Super Easy

PREDIABETIC DIET COOKBOOK

After 50

A Complete Low-Carb, Low-Sugar Action Plan to Manage and Reverse Pre-Diabetes and Prevent Diabetes

Alina Cobb

Prediabetes Meal Plan and Shopping Guide

Disclaimer

The information provided in this book, "Super Easy Prediabetic Diet Cookbook After 50: A Complete Low-Carb, Low-Sugar Action Plan to Manage and Reverse Pre-Diabetes and Prevent Diabetes" is for educational and informational purposes only. It is not intended as a substitute for professional medical advice or treatment. Always seek the advice of your physician or other qualified healthcare provider with any questions regarding a medical condition.

While we have made every effort to ensure the accuracy and completeness of the content, we do not guarantee the reliability, suitability, or effectiveness of the recipes, suggestions, or dietary guidelines presented herein. The author, publisher, and contributors are not liable for any personal injury, damage, or loss arising from the use of the information presented in this book. Readers are responsible for their own health and should consult with a healthcare professional before making any dietary or lifestyle changes. The recipes and meal plans in this book are intended to promote healthy aging and well-being, but individual results may vary.

It's important to consult with a qualified healthcare professional or nutritionist before making significant changes to your diet or lifestyle, especially if you have existing health conditions, allergies, or dietary restrictions.

The recipes and dietary recommendations in this book are based on general principles of nutrition and healthy eating. Individual nutritional needs may vary, and what works well for one person may not be suitable for another.

We disclaim any liability for any loss, injury, or damage incurred as a result of the use or misuse of the information provided in this book. Readers are encouraged to use their own judgment and discretion when applying the content to their personal dietary and health practices.

By using this book, you agree that you are responsible for your own health decisions and understand that the information provided is not a substitute for professional medical advice or treatment. Always seek the advice of a qualified healthcare provider with any questions or concerns you may have regarding your health or dietary needs.

CONTENTS

Chapter 1: Introduction   06

- Pre-Diabetes Management After 50
- Diagnosing Pre-Diabetes

Chapter 2: Prediabetes & Nutrition   12

- The Power of Balanced Nutrition
- Creating a Balanced Plate
- Meal Planning

Chapter 3: Breakfast and Brunch   20

- Spinach and Mushroom Frittata
- Chia Seed Pudding with Berries
- Avocado Toast with Poached Egg
- Greek Yogurt Parfait with Nuts and Seeds
- Quinoa Breakfast Bowl
- Sweet Potato Hash
- Berry Almond Smoothie
- Greek Yogurt and Berry Parfait
- Oatmeal with Walnuts and Pear
- Veggie Scramble with Avocado
- Almond Flour Pancakes with Blueberry Sauce
- Tomato and Zucchini Omelette
- Cottage Cheese and Peach Bowl
- Kale and White Bean Breakfast Sauté
- Broccoli and Cheese Egg Muffins
- Cinnamon Almond Porridge
- Smoked Salmon and Avocado Wrap
- Mediterranean Veggie Omelette
- Pumpkin Seed and Almond Yogurt
- Avocado and Egg Breakfast Salad

Chapter 4: Vegetarian Mains & Sides   41

- Quinoa and Black Bean Stuffed Peppers
- Lentil and Mushroom Shepherd's Pie
- Roasted Cauliflower and Chickpea Curry
- Zucchini Noodles with Pesto and Cherry Tomatoes
- Eggplant and Tofu Stir-Fry
- Balsamic Roasted Brussels Sprouts
- Stuffed Acorn Squash with Quinoa and Cranberries

- Lemon Garlic Roasted Asparagus
- Barley and Roasted Vegetable Pilaf
- Spaghetti Squash Primavera
- Chickpea and Spinach Curry

Chapter 5: Soup and Stew   53

- Lentil Vegetable Soup
- Tomato and White Bean Stew
- Chicken and Barley Soup
- Autumn Bisque
- Greens and Beans Turkey Soup
- Butternut Squash and Apple Soup
- Chicken and Vegetable Soup
- Spinach and White Bean Soup

Chapter 6: Meatless Main Dishes   62

- Zucchini Noodles with Pesto
- Lentil and Vegetable Stir-Fry
- Chickpea and Spinach Curry
- Eggplant and Tomato Stew
- Cauliflower and Chickpea Tacos
- Spaghetti Squash Pad Thai
- Mediterranean Chickpea Salad
- Eggplant Parmesan
- Caprese Salad
- Caprese Stuffed Portobello Mushrooms
- Vegetable Paella

Chapter 7: Chicken and Turkey   74

- Avocado and Turkey Wrap
- Chicken and Spinach Stuffed Portobello Mushrooms
- Turkey and Lentil Stuffed Bell Peppers
- Lemon Garlic Roast Chicken Thighs
- Chicken and Spinach Alfredo Pasta
- Turkey and Quinoa Stuffed Bell Peppers
- Lemon Herb Roasted Chicken Breast
- Turkey and Vegetable Stir-Fry
- Grilled Lemon Herb Turkey Cutlets
- Chicken and Quinoa Salad with Lemon Vinaigrette
- Turkey and Vegetable Skewers
- Lemon Garlic Chicken and Broccoli Stir-Fry
- Mediterranean Turkey Meatballs with Zucchini Noodles

Chapter 8: Beef, Pork, & Lamb — 88

- Lamb Curry with Cauliflower Rice
- Beef and Vegetable Stir-Fry with Quinoa
- Pork Chops with Balsamic Glaze
- Grilled Lamb Chops with Mint Chimichurri
- Pork Tenderloin with Maple Glaze
- Beef Stir-Fry with Broccoli and Brown Rice
- Pork Tenderloin with Roasted Vegetables
- Lamb and Chickpea Curry
- Beef and Vegetable Skewers with Quinoa
- Pork and Bean Chili

Chapter 9: Fish & Seafood — 99

- Creamy Garlic Shrimp Pasta
- Lemon Herb Baked Cod
- Spicy Grilled Shrimp Tacos
- Coconut Lime Shrimp Curry
- Mediterranean Grilled Swordfish
- Grilled Salmon with Lemon Herb Butter
- Shrimp and Avocado Salad
- Baked Cod with Roasted Vegetables
- Lemon Garlic Herb Grilled Shrimp
- Baked Lemon Herb Tilapia

Chapter 10: Sauce, Dips & Dressings — 110

- Spicy Sriracha Mayo
- Creamy Garlic Parmesan Dip
- Avocado Lime Dressing
- Tangy Honey Mustard Dip
- Lemon Herb Yogurt Sauce
- Creamy Cilantro Lime Dressing
- Avocado Yogurt Dip
- Tangy Balsamic Vinaigrette
- Roasted Red Pepper Hummus

Chapter 11: Smoothies — 120

- Berry Bliss Delight
- Tropical Turmeric Delight
- Spinach Berry Blast
- Cinnamon Apple Pie Delight
- Berry Avocado Powerhouse
- Tropical Mango Tango
- Chocolate Peanut Butter Bliss
- Green Power Smoothie
- Berry Blast Smoothie
- Tropical Paradise Smoothie
- Almond Butter Banana Smoothie

Chapter 12: Family Dinner — 132

- Coconut-Crusted Baked Tilapia
- Quinoa Stuffed Bell Peppers
- Veggie Hummus Wrap
- Asian Chicken Noodle Soup
- Garlic Herb Grilled Halibut
- Shrimp and Avocado Salad
- Pan-Seared Tuna Steak with Lemon Herb Butter
- Grilled Lemon Herb Chicken with Quinoa and Steamed Broccoli
- Baked Salmon with Asparagus and Brown Rice
- Spaghetti Squash with Tomato Basil Sauce

Chapter 13: Prediabetes Meal Plan and Grocery List — 143

- Week 1 Prediabetes Meal Plan
- Week 2 Prediabetes Meal Plan
- Week 3 Prediabetes Meal Plan
- Prediabetes Meal Plan Shopping Guide and Grocery List

Appendix — 149

- Appendix 1: The 2024 Dirty Dozen™ and Clean Fifteen™
- Appendix 2: Measurement Conversions
- Appendix 3: Recipe Index

Chapter One

Introduction

Picture this: a bustling kitchen filled with the tantalizing aromas of sizzling spices and wholesome ingredients, a sanctuary where every meal is not just a nourishing delight but a crucial step toward reclaiming your vitality, overcoming cravings, and transforming your relationship with food. This is the heart of this book. My name is Alina Cobb, and I am more than just an author; I am a dedicated healthcare professional who has witnessed the silent struggles of diabetes firsthand. Every week, I meet individuals who, unbeknownst to them, have been living with prediabetes or diabetes for years. Their stories are not mere statistics; they are real people facing the daunting challenges and emotional toll that come with unmanaged diabetes.

I have seen the worry in their eyes as they grapple with the reality of their health condition, and I have felt their determination to make meaningful changes. These encounters have profoundly inspired me to create this cookbook, a beacon of hope and practicality for those over 50 who are ready to take control of their health.

"Super Easy Prediabetic Diet Cookbook After 50" is more than a collection of recipes; it is an invitation to embark on a new chapter of your life. A chapter where every meal is an opportunity to nourish your body, delight your senses, and empower yourself with the knowledge and confidence to manage your health. Together, let's turn your kitchen into a haven of wellness, one delicious recipe at a time.

Pre–Diabetes Decoded: Understanding and Managing Your Blood Sugar

If you're holding this cookbook, you're likely concerned about pre-diabetes, either for yourself or a loved one. A pre-diabetes diagnosis can be a wake-up call, signaling the need for immediate action. Understanding pre-diabetes and taking proactive steps can help you manage and even reverse it. By choosing this cookbook, you're already taking a crucial step towards reclaiming your health and preventing type 2 diabetes.

To understand pre-diabetes, you first need to know the basics of diabetes. Diabetes mellitus, or diabetes, affects how your body handles glucose, the sugar from your food. Insulin, a hormone, helps move glucose into your cells for energy. In diabetes, the body either doesn't produce enough insulin or can't use it properly, causing high blood sugar levels.

There are different types of diabetes, but our focus here is primarily on type 2 diabetes, which accounts for the majority of diabetes cases. In type 2 diabetes, the pancreas still produces insulin, but not enough, or the body becomes resistant to its effects. This type is often linked to factors like obesity, lack of exercise, and a sedentary lifestyle.

Type 1 diabetes, on the other hand, is less common and typically diagnosed at a younger age. It's an autoimmune condition where the body's immune system attacks the insulin-producing cells in the pancreas. Individuals with type 1 diabetes require lifelong insulin therapy.

Gestational diabetes occurs during pregnancy, affecting how insulin works due to hormonal changes. While it usually resolves after childbirth, women who have had gestational diabetes are at higher risk of developing type 2 diabetes later in life, especially if they maintain an unhealthy weight or lifestyle.

It's crucial to note that while diabetes can be managed, it currently has no cure. Proper diet, regular exercise, and medication may be necessary to control blood sugar levels. Pre-diabetes is a warning sign that should not be ignored, as it can progress to type 2 diabetes if left untreated. This cookbook aims to provide you with practical guidance and delicious recipes to support a healthy lifestyle and manage pre-diabetes effectively.

Type 2 Diabetes

Now, let's delve into the specifics of type 2 diabetes to gain a deeper understanding. Type 2 diabetes's roots lie in how our bodies utilize sugar as fuel. Our fuel sources, including sugar, fat, and protein, can be converted into sugar and transported through the bloodstream. When sugar intake exceeds requirements, it can lead to a condition akin to a repetitive stress injury, eventually culminating in type 2 diabetes.

At the cellular level, type 2 diabetes disrupts the delicate balance of nutrient intake, waste elimination, and oxygen delivery. This condition manifests as elevated blood sugar levels and insulin sensitivity issues. Insulin, produced by the pancreas, acts as a key to open doors for glucose to enter cells. However, over time, excess fat in cells interferes with glucose entry, leading to insulin insensitivity.

Elevated blood sugar causes three primary problems:
1. **Sticky Blood:** Glucose buildup in the blood makes it sticky, hindering the function of hormones and other substances traveling in the bloodstream.
2. **Capillary Clogging:** Sticky blood can clog capillaries, impairing blood flow to vital areas of the body.
3. **Swelling and Water Retention:** High sugar levels bring water into cells and surrounding areas, causing swelling that further restricts cell function and circulation.

These effects initiate a cascade of damage, resulting in nerve damage, vision deterioration, kidney problems, and compromised immune function. Diabetics are more susceptible to infections due to impaired cell function, blood protein dysfunction, and compromised immune response caused by sticky blood and swelling.

The implications of type 2 diabetes extend beyond physical health issues like cardiovascular disease and circulatory problems. Recent events, such as the COVID-19 pandemic, have highlighted the vulnerability of diabetics, emphasizing the critical importance of managing blood sugar levels and adopting a healthy lifestyle.

This cookbook serves as a comprehensive guide, offering practical guidance and delectable recipes to support a healthy lifestyle and effectively manage pre-diabetes. Let's embark on this journey together, empowering ourselves with knowledge and actionable steps to navigate the complexities of diabetes and enhance our overall well-being.

Pre–Diabetes Management After 50

Managing pre-diabetes becomes especially crucial after the age of 50 due to several key factors that influence health and well-being during this stage of life.

1. **Increased Risk of Type 2 Diabetes:** As individuals age, their risk of developing type 2 diabetes naturally increases. Pre-diabetes serves as a warning sign that the body is struggling to regulate blood sugar levels effectively. Without intervention, pre-diabetes can progress to type 2 diabetes, which can lead to serious health complications such as heart disease, stroke, kidney disease, and nerve damage.
2. **Metabolic Changes:** Aging is often accompanied by changes in metabolism. Hormonal fluctuations, decreased muscle mass, and changes in fat distribution can affect how the body processes glucose. This can contribute to insulin resistance, a hallmark of pre-diabetes and type 2 diabetes.
3. **Reduced Physical Activity:** Many individuals may become less physically active as they age, which can exacerbate insulin resistance and lead to weight gain. Lack of regular exercise can also impact overall metabolic health and increase the risk of developing diabetes.
4. **Age-Related Health Conditions:** Older adults are more likely to have other health conditions such as high blood pressure, high cholesterol, and cardiovascular disease, which are often linked to diabetes. Managing pre-diabetes effectively can help reduce the risk of complications from these concurrent health issues.

5. Slower Healing: Aging can slow down the body's healing processes, making it more challenging to recover from injuries or illnesses related to diabetes. Managing pre-diabetes can help maintain overall health and resilience in the face of potential health challenges.

6. Quality of Life: Effective management of pre-diabetes can significantly improve quality of life for individuals over 50. It can help maintain energy levels, prevent diabetes-related complications, and support overall well-being and longevity.

7. Family History: Family history plays a significant role in diabetes risk. Individuals with a family history of diabetes, especially if diagnosed after the age of 50, should be particularly vigilant about managing pre-diabetes to reduce their risk of developing type 2 diabetes.

Managing pre-diabetes after the age of 50 is crucial due the potential impact on overall quality of life. It's essential for individuals in this age group to prioritize healthy lifestyle habits, regular monitoring of blood sugar levels, and working closely with healthcare professionals to prevent or delay the onset of diabetes and its associated complications.

Diagnosing Prediabetes

Prediabetes often lurks silently without noticeable symptoms, leaving many unaware of their condition. However, certain subtle signs may hint at prediabetes. According to the American Academy of Dermatology Association, individuals with prediabetes may develop acanthosis nigricans, characterized by darkened skin around the neck and armpits, and small skin tags in areas like the eyes, neck, groin, and armpits. These skin changes stem from elevated blood sugar and insulin levels in the body.

Since prediabetes symptoms can be elusive, effective diagnosis requires close collaboration with your medical team. Your healthcare providers can assess your risk based on family history, medical background, and lifestyle choices. It's crucial to advocate for your health by honestly evaluating your physical activity levels and dietary habits. Regular screenings are beneficial, especially if your lifestyle leans towards low physical activity, lacks fruits and vegetables, or includes high amounts of processed foods and sugars.

The National Institute of Diabetes and Digestive and Kidney Diseases recommends three primary screening tests for prediabetes: A1C, fasting plasma glucose, and a two-hour post 75g oral glucose challenge.

- **A1C Test:** This simple blood test assesses long-term blood glucose management without requiring fasting. It measures average blood sugar levels over the past two to three months, providing valuable insights into your overall glucose control.
- **Fasting Plasma Glucose Test:** Conducted through a blood sample after an eight-hour fasting period (except for water), this test evaluates your blood sugar levels in a fasting state. It's best done early in the morning for accurate results.
- **Two-Hour Post 75g Oral Glucose Challenge:** This test involves drinking a sweet solution, followed by blood sugar measurements two hours later. It helps doctors gauge how effectively your body processes glucose.

Elevated results in any of these tests can indicate prediabetes, prompting further evaluation and proactive measures to manage your condition effectively. By staying proactive with screenings and maintaining open communication with your healthcare team, you can take charge of your health and address prediabetes before it progresses to type 2 diabetes.

Chapter Two

Prediabetes and Nutrition

Embarking on a journey to reverse prediabetes through healthy nutrition doesn't have to feel daunting or unattainable. The beauty of adopting a healthy diet lies in its simplicity, flexibility, and the transformative power it holds for your well-being. In this chapter, we'll delve into the practical and delicious ways you can use food to reverse prediabetes and nourish your body.

The Power of Balanced Nutrition

What we eat plays a crucial role in our blood sugar levels and overall risk of developing prediabetes. Our bodies thrive on a balanced intake of micronutrients (vitamins and minerals) and macronutrients (carbohydrates, fats, and proteins). Each of these elements serves a unique purpose in supporting our health and vitality.

Carbohydrates: Often misunderstood, carbohydrates are essential for providing energy to our central nervous system, including our brain. They fuel our muscles, support bodily functions, and provide fiber, a key component found in fruits and vegetables. Fiber promotes healthy digestion, keeps you feeling full and satisfied after meals, and helps maintain stable blood sugar levels and regular bowel movements.

Fats: Contrary to popular belief, fats are not the enemy. They serve as a valuable source of energy, aid in the absorption of vitamins and hormone production, and help regulate body temperature. Including healthy fats in your diet is crucial for overall well-being.

Proteins: Vital for growth, maintenance, and repair of the body, proteins are the building blocks of life. They play a significant role in hormone and immune health, ensuring your body functions optimally.

Creating a Balanced Plate

Achieving a healthy diet involves incorporating all three macronutrients into your meals. Rather than focusing on restriction, the key is to embrace variety and balance. Here are some practical tips to guide your journey towards healthy nutrition for prediabetes reversal:

1. **Embrace Plant-Based Foods:** Incorporate a variety of colorful fruits, vegetables, whole grains, legumes, nuts, and seeds into your meals. These plant-based foods are rich in fiber, vitamins, and minerals, promoting overall health and helping manage blood sugar levels.
2. **Mindful Eating:** Practice mindful eating by paying attention to hunger cues, savoring each bite, and eating slowly. This allows you to enjoy your food, prevents overeating, and fosters a positive relationship with food.
3. **Portion Control:** Be mindful of portion sizes to avoid excessive calorie intake. Use smaller plates, measure servings, and listen to your body's signals of fullness.
4. **Hydration:** Drink plenty of water throughout the day to stay hydrated and support overall health.
5. **Limit Processed Foods:** Minimize consumption of processed foods, sugary beverages, and high-fat snacks. Opt for whole, nutrient-dense foods instead.

By implementing these practical nutrition changes into your daily routine, you'll not only support prediabetes reversal but also enhance your overall health and well-being. Remember, it's about progress, not perfection. Each healthy choice you make brings you closer to a healthier, happier you.

Prediabetes Reversal – Understanding the Role of Carbs

Carbohydrates often get a bad rap in the world of nutrition, but the truth is, they play a vital role in our health, especially when it comes to managing prediabetes. Let's dive deeper into understanding the different types of carbs and how they impact our bodies.

Carbohydrates are essentially sugar molecules linked together. Natural sugars found in carbohydrates are not inherently unhealthy; in fact, they provide essential support for our cell structures and serve as fuel for our brains and bodies. The misconception that carbs are the enemy stems from a lack of distinction between complex and simple carbohydrates.

Complex Carbs: The Heroes

Complex carbohydrates are the superheroes of the carb world. They include fruits, vegetables, and whole grains, all rich in fiber. Fiber slows down digestion and absorption, leading to better insulin function and balanced blood sugar levels. Think of complex carbs as your body's best friend, supporting overall health and well-being.

Simple Carbs: The Villains

On the flip side, we have simple carbohydrates, often laden with added sugars. These include refined sugars like white sugar, corn syrup, and honey. Simple carbs are rapidly digested and absorbed, causing sugar spikes and potentially leading to insulin resistance and prediabetes if consumed excessively.

Choosing Healthy Carbs

The key to harnessing the power of carbs for prediabetes reversal lies in focusing on healthy sources. Here are some tips to guide your carb choices:

1. **Load Up on Veggies and Fruits**: Non-starchy vegetables and fruits should be staples in your meals. They are rich in antioxidants, vitamins, minerals, and fiber, offering a plethora of health benefits.
2. **Opt for Whole Grains**: Choose whole grains like whole-wheat pasta, brown rice, quinoa, and barley. These grains provide more nutrients and fiber compared to their refined counterparts, supporting stable blood sugar levels.

3. Include Legumes: Beans, lentils, and peas are not only excellent sources of protein but also healthy carbohydrates. They contribute to satiety, promote digestive health, and help regulate blood sugar.

4. Mind Your Portions: While whole grains are beneficial, portion control is key. Stick to appropriate serving sizes to maintain balanced carbohydrate intake.

By making these simple yet impactful changes to your diet, you can harness the power of healthy carbs to support prediabetes reversal and overall well-being. Remember, it's about making informed choices and finding what works best for your body and lifestyle.

Meal Planning

Have you ever noticed that even the best planners sometimes overlook planning their meals? It's a curious phenomenon. Many people excel at planning in various aspects of their lives but often neglect to plan what or when they will eat. Perhaps it's because food is so readily available that it seems unnecessary to plan. Some may even believe that healthy eating is all about willpower. However, I assure you that successful meal planning has little to do with willpower and everything to do with informed choices and preparation.

The Importance of Meal Planning

Every time you eat or drink presents an opportunity to nourish your body. What you consume in the short term affects your energy levels, comfort, mood, and productivity. Over time, your food choices significantly impact your long-term well-being, influencing your risks of developing conditions like type 2 diabetes and dementia. Given the importance of nutrition, meal planning becomes a crucial aspect of maintaining a healthy lifestyle.

Overcoming Common Barriers to Meal Planning

Many individuals face barriers to meal planning, often due to a lack of awareness of its benefits. However, understanding and addressing these barriers can lead to better nutrition, improved health outcomes, and reduced stress. Here are some common obstacles and their solutions:

1. **Time Constraint:** While meal planning requires initial time investment, it ultimately saves time in the long run. Once you create a meal planning routine, you can reuse previous plans and streamline the process.
2. **Diverse Preferences:** Balancing varied tastes within a household can be challenging. Involving family members in meal planning and accommodating their preferences can foster harmony. Pair less favored foods with favorites to ensure everyone finds something enjoyable.
3. **Conflicting Schedules:** Busy schedules often disrupt meal times. Incorporating schedule considerations into your meal plan can help. Simple meals like leftovers or easy-to-prepare dishes accommodate hectic days without compromising nutrition.
4. **Unexpected Events:** Unforeseen circumstances may disrupt plans. Maintaining a backup meal plan and stocking essentials in your kitchen can help you whip up quick and healthy meals, avoiding reliance on unhealthy fast food options.
5. **Lack of Cooking Knowledge:** Not knowing what constitutes a healthy meal or lacking cooking ideas can be addressed through education and recipe collections. This book provides guidance on nutritious meal options and encourages creating a repertoire of go-to recipes.

By acknowledging these barriers and implementing practical solutions, you can embrace meal planning as a tool for promoting better nutrition, reducing waste, saving time, and enhancing overall well-being. Remember, meal planning is a skill that improves with practice and can significantly benefit your health and lifestyle.

Plate Method for Meal Planning

The Plate Method simplifies meal planning into three easy steps, making it an effective tool for crafting balanced and prediabetes-friendly meals. Let's delve deeper into this method to understand how it can guide your meal choices effortlessly.

Step 1: Divide Your Plate

Begin with a 9-inch plate and imagine drawing a line down the middle, creating two equal halves.

Step 2: Fill Your Plate

- Nonstarchy Vegetables (½ plate): Allocate half of your plate to nonstarchy vegetables, which may amount to 1–2 cups of vegetables. Options include mixed greens, kale, cucumber, broccoli, and more.
- Starchy Foods (¼ plate): Use a quarter of your plate for starchy foods like sweet potatoes, lentils, brown rice, or pasta, ranging from ½ to 1 cup.
- Protein-Rich Foods (¼ plate): The remaining quarter is for protein-rich foods such as salmon, chicken, tofu, or beans, around 3–4 ounces or ¾–1 cup diced.

Optional Additions:

Include a piece of fruit the size of a tennis ball, a serving of dairy, or both, for added nutrition.

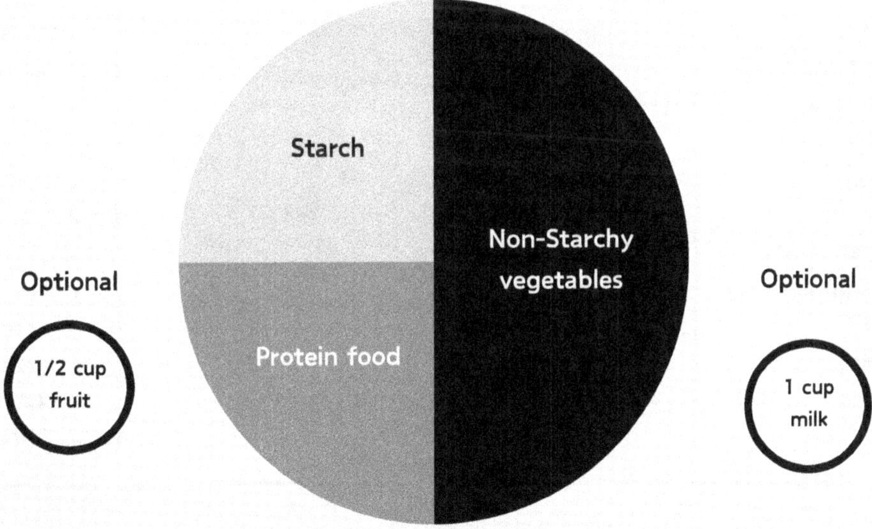

Table 1: Food options for prediabetes–friendly meals

Starchy foods	Protein-rich foods	Non-starchy vegetables
• Sweet potatoes • Quinoa • Brown rice • Wild rice • Barley • Bulgur • Steel-cut oats • Rolled oats • Buckwheat • Farro • Spelt • Millet • Amaranth • Sorghum • Freekeh • Whole grain bread • Whole grain pasta • Lentils • Chickpeas • Black beans • Kidney beans • Navy beans • Pinto beans • Green peas • Corn • Butternut squash • Acorn squash • Pumpkin • Plantains • Parsnips	• Skinless chicken breast • Turkey breast • Lean cuts of beef (e.g.sirloin or tenderloin) • Lean cuts of pork (e.g. loin or tenderloin) • Fish (e.g. salmon, tuna, and cod) • Shellfish (e.g. shrimp, crab, and lobster) • Eggs • Egg whites • Greek yogurt (unsweetened) • Cottage cheese (low-fat) • Tofu • Tempeh • Edamame • Lentils • Chickpeas • Black beans • Kidney beans • Navy beans • Quinoa • Chia seeds • Flaxseeds • Hemp seeds • Pumpkin seeds • Sunflower seeds • Almonds • Walnuts • Peanuts • Pistachios • Cashews • Low-fat cheese (e.g. mozzarella or ricotta)	• Spinach • Kale • Broccoli • Cauliflower • Brussels sprouts • Asparagus • Bell peppers • Zucchini • Cucumber • Green beans • Lettuce • Cabbage • Swiss chard • Collard greens • Bok choy • Radishes • Arugula • Celery • Mushrooms • Tomatoes • Eggplant • Onions • Leeks • Garlic • Okra • Turnips • Fennel • Endive • Artichokes • Snow peas

The Beauty of the Plate Method

This method provides clarity on what and how much to eat, ensuring a balanced meal without the need for calorie or carb counting. Adjust portions based on hunger, especially focusing on nonstarchy vegetables for satiety as they are low in calories and carbohydrates.

Adapting to Bowls

While the Plate Method emphasizes using a plate, it's flexible enough to apply to bowls as well. Follow these guidelines:

- Allocate equal volumes of starchy food and protein-rich food.
- Ensure nonstarchy vegetables make up at least half of your meal for optimal nutrition and satiety.

Making Meal Planning Simple

Here are five steps to perfect your meal planning using the Plate Method:

1. **Look Ahead:** Consider your schedule, family preferences, and quick-to-prepare options for busy days.
2. **Plan Your Meals:** Use a calendar or template to jot down planned dinners, ensuring a balance of protein, starch, and nonstarchy vegetables.
3. **Take Inventory:** Create a grocery list based on your planned meals, adding any needed ingredients.
4. **Be Flexible:** Allow room for adjustments based on specials or new recipe ideas.
5. **Reuse Menus:** Recycle successful menus to streamline future meal planning efforts.

Once you grasp the Plate Method's basics, unleash your creativity. Mix and match protein-rich foods with nonstarchy vegetables and grains to create diverse and satisfying meals. Refer to the provided examples for inspiration and enjoy balanced, prediabetes-friendly eating without the guesswork.

Chapter Three

Breakfast and Brunch

Starting your day with a nutritious meal is essential, especially when managing pre-diabetes. In this chapter, "Breakfast and Brunch Recipes for Pre-Diabetic Diet," you'll find delicious and balanced recipes designed to keep your blood sugar levels stable while providing the energy you need to tackle your day.

For those over 50, maintaining a healthy diet becomes even more crucial as metabolism slows down and nutritional needs change. The recipes in this chapter focus on high-fiber, low-glycemic ingredients, and lean proteins that not only help manage blood sugar but also support overall health and well-being.

Whether you're craving a hearty breakfast or a light brunch, these recipes will inspire you to make healthier choices without sacrificing flavor. From protein-packed egg dishes to fiber-rich whole grains and fresh vegetables, you'll discover a variety of meals that are both satisfying and beneficial for managing pre-diabetes. Let's embark on this culinary journey and transform the most important meal of the day into a delightful and health-boosting experience.

SPINACH AND MUSHROOM FRITTATA

A hearty and nutritious frittata packed with protein and fiber to start
your day without spiking your blood sugar.

Servings: 2 Prep Time: 10 minutes Cook Time: 20 minutes Carbs per Serving: 8g

INGREDIENTS

- 4 large eggs
- 1 cup fresh spinach, chopped
- 1/2 cup mushrooms, sliced
- 1/4 cup onions, diced
- 1/4 cup low-fat feta cheese
- 1 tbsp olive oil
- Salt and pepper to taste

DIRECTIONS

1. Preheat the oven to 375°F (190°C).
2. In a skillet, heat olive oil over medium heat. Sauté onions and mushrooms until tender.
3. Add spinach and cook until wilted.
4. In a bowl, whisk eggs, salt, and pepper. Pour over the vegetables in the skillet.
5. Sprinkle feta cheese on top.
6. Transfer the skillet to the oven and bake for 15 minutes or until the eggs are set.

Nutrient Content (per serving):
- Calories: 220
- Total Fat: 16g
- Protein: 14g
- Carbohydrates: 8g
- Sugars: 3g
- Fiber: 2g
- Sodium: 340mg

"Every meal is a chance to heal."

INGREDIENT TIPS:
- Spinach has a low glycemic index and is rich in fiber, which helps in managing blood sugar levels.
- Mushrooms provide a savory flavor with minimal impact on glucose levels.

CHIA SEED PUDDING WITH BERRIES

A refreshing and filling pudding that's perfect for a quick breakfast or a sweet brunch treat, keeping your blood sugar in check.

Servings: 1 Prep   Time: 15 minutes (plus overnight soaking)   Cook Time: 0 minutes

Carbs per Serving: 20g

INGREDIENTS

- 3 tbsp chia seeds
- 1 cup unsweetened almond milk
- 1/2 cup mixed berries (strawberries, blueberries, raspberries)
- 1 tbsp almond slivers
- 1 tsp vanilla extract
- Stevia to taste

DIRECTIONS

1. In a jar, mix chia seeds with almond milk and vanilla extract.
2. Sweeten with stevia to taste.
3. Let the mixture sit overnight in the refrigerator.
4. Top with fresh berries and almond slivers before serving.

Nutrient Content (per serving):

- Calories: 300
- Total Fat: 18g
- Protein: 8g
- Carbohydrates: 20g
- Sugars: 5g
- Fiber: 10g
- Sodium: 180mg

"Nourish your body, nurture your soul."

INGREDIENT TIPS:

- Chia seeds are high in fiber and omega-3 fatty acids, which can help regulate blood sugar levels.
- Berries are low on the glycemic index and add natural sweetness without a significant sugar spike.

AVOCADO TOAST WITH POACHED EGG

Savory avocado toast topped with a perfectly poached egg for a balanced meal that's both delicious and diabetes-friendly.

Servings: 1 Prep Time: 5 minutes Cook Time: 10 minutes Carbs per Serving: 15g

INGREDIENTS

- 1 slice whole-grain bread
- 1/2 ripe avocado
- 1 egg
- 1 tsp lemon juice
- Salt and pepper to taste
- Chili flakes (optional)

DIRECTIONS

1. Toast the whole-grain bread to your liking.
2. Mash the avocado with lemon juice, salt, and pepper.
3. Spread the avocado mixture on the toast.
4. Poach the egg and place it on top of the avocado toast.
5. Sprinkle with chili flakes for added flavor.

Nutrient Content (per serving):

- Calories: 330
- Total Fat: 23g
- Protein: 13g
- Carbohydrates: 15g
- Sugars: 2g
- Fiber: 7g
- Sodium: 320mg

"Healthy eating is a journey, not a destination."

INGREDIENT TIPS:

- Avocado is a great source of monounsaturated fats and has a low glycemic index.
- Whole-grain bread provides complex carbohydrates that are digested slowly, preventing blood sugar spikes.

GREEK YOGURT PARFAIT WITH NUTS AND SEEDS

A creamy and crunchy parfait that's not only tasty but also stabilizes your blood sugar levels throughout the morning.

Servings: 1 Prep Time: 5 minutes Cook Time: 0 minutes Carbs per Serving: 18g

INGREDIENTS

- 3/4 cup plain Greek yogurt
- 1/4 cup granola (low-sugar)
- 2 tbsp mixed nuts (walnuts, almonds, pistachios)
- 1 tbsp pumpkin seeds
- 1 tbsp sunflower seeds
- Cinnamon to taste

DIRECTIONS

1. Layer Greek yogurt at the bottom of a glass or bowl.
2. Add a layer of granola, then sprinkle with nuts and seeds.
3. Repeat the layers if desired.
4. Top with a dash of cinnamon for flavor.

Nutrient Content (per serving):
- Calories: 350
- Total Fat: 20g
- Protein: 25g
- Carbohydrates: 18g
- Sugars: 6g
- Fiber: 4g
- Sodium: 65mg

"Small changes can make a big difference."

INGREDIENT TIPS:
- Greek yogurt is high in protein and low in carbohydrates, making it an excellent choice for blood sugar management.
- Nuts and seeds add healthy fats and fiber, which can help slow down the absorption of sugars.

QUINOA BREAKFAST BOWL

A warm and comforting breakfast bowl with the perfect balance of protein, fiber, and complex carbs to maintain steady glucose levels.

Servings: 2 Prep Time: 5 minutes Cook Time: 15 minutes Carbs per Serving: 30g

---

INGREDIENTS

- 1/2 cup quinoa
- 1 cup water
- 1/2 cup almond milk
- 1 apple, diced
- 1/4 cup raisins
- 1/4 tsp cinnamon
- 1 tbsp honey (optional)

DIRECTIONS

1. Rinse quinoa under cold water.
2. In a pot, bring water to a boil. Add quinoa and reduce heat to simmer.
3. Cook until quinoa is fluffy and water is absorbed, about 15 minutes.
4. Stir in almond milk, diced apple, raisins, and cinnamon.
5. Sweeten with honey if desired.

Nutrient Content (per serving):
- Calories: 250
- Total Fat: 4g
- Protein: 8g
- Carbohydrates: 30g
- Sugars: 13g
- Fiber: 5g
- Sodium: 30mg

"Invest in your health, it pays the best interest."

INGREDIENT TIPS:
- Quinoa is a complete protein and has a low glycemic index, making it a smart carb choice.
- Apples and raisins provide natural sweetness and fiber, which aids in blood sugar control.

SWEET POTATO HASH

A colorful and satisfying hash that combines the natural sweetness of sweet potatoes with savory peppers and onions.

Servings: 2 Prep Time: 10 minutes Cook Time: 20 minutes Carbs per Serving: 30g

INGREDIENTS

- 1 large sweet potato, peeled and diced
- 1 red bell pepper, chopped
- 1 small red onion, diced
- 2 cloves garlic, minced
- 2 tbsp olive oil
- 1 tsp smoked paprika
- Salt and pepper to taste
- Fresh parsley for garnish

DIRECTIONS

1. Heat olive oil in a skillet over medium heat.
2. Add diced sweet potato, red bell pepper, and red onion. Sauté until tender.
3. Stir in minced garlic, smoked paprika, salt, and pepper.
4. Cook for an additional 5 minutes until flavors meld.
5. Garnish with fresh parsley before serving.

Nutrient Content (per serving):
- Calories: 280
- Total Fat: 10g
- Protein: 4g
- Carbohydrates: 30g
- Sugars: 8g
- Fiber: 6g
- Sodium: 180mg

"You are what you eat, so eat something sweet... for your body!"

INGREDIENT TIPS:
- Sweet potatoes have a lower glycemic index than regular potatoes and are rich in vitamins and fiber.
- Red bell peppers add color, flavor, and vitamin C.

BERRY ALMOND SMOOTHIE

A refreshing and creamy smoothie packed with antioxidants and essential nutrients to kickstart your day.

Servings: 1 Prep Time: 5 minutes Cook Time: 0 minutes Carbs per Serving: 25g

---

INGREDIENTS

- 1 cup unsweetened almond milk
- 1/2 cup mixed berries (blueberries, raspberries, strawberries)
- 1 tbsp almond butter
- 1 tbsp chia seeds
- Ice cubes (optional)

DIRECTIONS

1. Blend almond milk, mixed berries, almond butter, and chia seeds until smooth.
2. Add ice cubes if desired for a colder texture.
3. Serve immediately.

Nutrient Content (per serving):

- Calories: 220
- Total Fat: 12g
- Protein: 6g
- Carbohydrates: 25g
- Sugars: 10g
- Fiber: 8g
- Sodium: 180mg

"Good food choices are good investments."

INGREDIENT TIPS:

- Berries are low in sugar and high in antioxidants, making them a great choice for blood sugar control.
- Almond butter provides healthy fats and protein.

GREEK YOGURT AND BERRY PARFAIT

A creamy and satisfying parfait that combines the tanginess of Greek yogurt with the sweetness of berries and the crunch of nuts. Perfect for a quick breakfast or snack!

Servings: 1 Prep Time: 5 minutes Cook Time: 0 minutes Carbs per Serving: 20g

---

INGREDIENTS

- 3/4 cup plain Greek yogurt
- 1/2 cup mixed berries (blueberries, raspberries, strawberries)
- 1 tbsp chopped nuts (almonds, walnuts, or pecans)
- 1 tbsp ground flaxseed
- 1 tsp honey (optional)

DIRECTIONS

1. Layer Greek yogurt at the bottom of a glass or bowl.
2. Add a layer of mixed berries.
3. Sprinkle chopped nuts and ground flaxseed on top.
4. Drizzle with honey if desired.
5. Repeat the layers if you prefer a larger portion.

Nutrient Content (per serving):
- Calories: 250
- Total Fat: 12g
- Protein: 15g
- Carbohydrates: 20g
- Sugars: 10g
- Fiber: 5g
- Sodium: 60mg

"Eat to live, not live to eat."

INGREDIENT TIPS:
- Greek yogurt provides protein and probiotics for gut health.
- Berries are rich in antioxidants and low in sugar.
- Nuts and flaxseed add healthy fats and fiber.

OATMEAL WITH WALNUTS AND PEAR

A warm and comforting bowl of oatmeal with the crunch of walnuts and sweetness of pear to start your day right.

Servings: 1 Prep Time: 5 minutes Cook Time: 10 minutes Carbs per Serving: 30g

INGREDIENTS

- 1/2 cup rolled oats
- 1 cup water or unsweetened almond milk
- 1 pear, diced
- 1/4 tsp cinnamon
- 1 tbsp walnuts, chopped
- 1 tsp chia seeds

DIRECTIONS

1. Bring water or almond milk to a boil in a pot.
2. Add oats and reduce heat to simmer, cooking for 5 minutes.
3. Stir in diced pear and cinnamon, cooking for another 5 minutes.
4. Serve topped with walnuts and chia seeds.

Nutrient Content (per serving):
- Calories: 270
- Total Fat: 8g
- Protein: 6g
- Carbohydrates: 30g
- Sugars: 10g
- Fiber: 7g
- Sodium: 5mg

"Your health is in your hands."

INGREDIENT TIPS:
- Oats are a great source of soluble fiber, which can help manage blood sugar levels.
- Pears provide natural sweetness and additional fiber.

VEGGIE SCRAMBLE WITH AVOCADO

A hearty and nutritious scramble that's quick to make and packed with flavors and textures to satisfy your morning hunger.

Servings: 1 Prep Time: 5 minutes Cook Time: 10 minutes Carbs per Serving: 15g

INGREDIENTS

- 2 large eggs
- 1/2 cup spinach, chopped
- 1/4 cup bell peppers, diced
- 1/4 avocado, sliced
- 1 tbsp olive oil
- Salt and pepper to taste

DIRECTIONS

1. Heat olive oil in a pan over medium heat.
2. Sauté bell peppers until soft.
3. Add spinach and cook until wilted.
4. Whisk eggs and pour into the pan, scrambling with the veggies.
5. Serve with sliced avocado on top.

Nutrient Content (per serving):
- Calories: 320
- Total Fat: 25g
- Protein: 14g
- Carbohydrates: 15g
- Sugars: 3g
- Fiber: 7g
- Sodium: 200mg

"Choose foods that love you back."

INGREDIENT TIPS:
- Eggs are a high-quality protein that can help keep you full and stabilize blood sugar.
- Avocado is full of healthy fats and fiber.

ALMOND FLOUR PANCAKES WITH BLUEBERRY SAUCE

Fluffy almond flour pancakes topped with a tangy blueberry sauce for a delightful breakfast that won't disrupt your glucose levels.

Servings: 2 Prep Time: 10 minutes Cook Time: 15 minutes Carbs per Serving: 20g

INGREDIENTS

- 1 cup almond flour
- 2 large eggs
- 1/4 cup unsweetened almond milk
- 1 tsp baking powder
- 1/2 cup blueberries
- 1 tbsp lemon juice
- Stevia to taste

DIRECTIONS

1. Mix almond flour, eggs, almond milk, and baking powder to form a batter.
2. Pour small amounts onto a heated non-stick pan, flipping when bubbles form.
3. For the sauce, heat blueberries and lemon juice in a saucepan until they break down into a sauce.
4. Sweeten with stevia to taste and serve over pancakes.

Nutrient Content (per serving):

- Calories: 280
- Total Fat: 22g
- Protein: 12g
- Carbohydrates: 20g
- Sugars: 5g
- Fiber: 5g
- Sodium: 300mg

"Eat well, feel well, live well."

INGREDIENT TIPS:

- Almond flour is a low-carb alternative to wheat flour and is rich in healthy fats.
- Blueberries are low-glycemic fruits that add natural sweetness without spiking blood sugar.

TOMATO AND ZUCCHINI OMELETTE

A fluffy omelette filled with fresh garden veggies and a touch of cheese for a satisfying and nutritious start to your day.

Servings: 1 Prep Time: 5 minutes Cook Time: 10 minutes Carbs per Serving: 10g

INGREDIENTS

- 2 large eggs
- 1/2 small zucchini, thinly sliced
- 1/2 tomato, diced
- 1 tbsp shredded low-fat cheese
- 1 tsp olive oil
- Salt and pepper to taste

DIRECTIONS

1. Beat the eggs in a bowl and season with salt and pepper.
2. Heat olive oil in a pan over medium heat.
3. Pour in the eggs and cook for a minute until they begin to set.
4. Place zucchini slices and tomato on one half of the omelette.
5. Sprinkle cheese over the vegetables.
6. Fold the omelette in half and cook until the cheese melts.

Nutrient Content (per serving):

- Calories: 220
- Total Fat: 15g
- Protein: 14g
- Carbohydrates: 10g
- Sugars: 6g
- Fiber: 2g
- Sodium: 210mg

"Healthy habits lead to healthy lives."

INGREDIENT TIPS:

- Zucchini is low in carbs and calories, making it ideal for blood sugar management.
- Tomatoes are rich in lycopene and vitamins, adding flavor and nutrition without spiking glucose levels.

COTTAGE CHEESE AND PEACH BOWL

A creamy and fruity bowl that's perfect for a light breakfast or snack, offering a good balance of protein and natural sugars.

Servings: 1 Prep Time: 5 minutes Cook Time: 0 minutes Carbs per Serving: 15g

INGREDIENTS

- 3/4 cup low-fat cottage cheese
- 1 medium peach, sliced
- 1 tbsp chopped pecans
- A sprinkle of cinnamon

DIRECTIONS

1. Place cottage cheese in a serving bowl.
2. Top with fresh peach slices and chopped pecans.
3. Dust with cinnamon for added flavor.

Nutrient Content (per serving):

- Calories: 200
- Total Fat: 8g
- Protein: 15g
- Carbohydrates: 15g
- Sugars: 12g
- Fiber: 2g
- Sodium: 350mg

"Make every bite count."

INGREDIENT TIPS:

- Cottage cheese is a great source of protein and calcium, which can help control hunger and blood sugar.
- Peaches add natural sweetness and are lower on the glycemic index compared to other fruits.

KALE AND WHITE BEAN BREAKFAST SAUTÉ

A hearty and healthy sauté that combines leafy greens with protein-rich beans for a filling and nutritious breakfast option.

Servings: 2 Prep Time: 10 minutes Cook Time: 15 minutes Carbs per Serving: 25g

INGREDIENTS

- 1 cup kale, chopped
- 1/2 cup white beans, cooked
- 1/4 cup cherry tomatoes, halved
- 2 cloves garlic, minced
- 2 tbsp olive oil
- Salt and pepper to taste
- Red pepper flakes (optional)

DIRECTIONS

1. Heat olive oil in a pan over medium heat.
2. Add garlic and sauté until fragrant.
3. Stir in kale and cook until slightly wilted.
4. Add white beans and cherry tomatoes, cooking until heated through.
5. Season with salt, pepper, and red pepper flakes if desired.

Nutrient Content (per serving):
- Calories: 250
- Total Fat: 14g
- Protein: 10g
- Carbohydrates: 25g
- Sugars: 2g
- Fiber: 6g
- Sodium: 400mg

"Fuel your body with goodness."

INGREDIENT TIPS:
- Kale is a nutrient-dense vegetable that's high in fiber and antioxidants.
- White beans are a good source of protein and have a low glycemic index, making them excellent for blood sugar control.

BROCCOLI AND CHEESE EGG MUFFINS

These egg muffins are a convenient and portable breakfast option, perfect for a quick bite on busy mornings.

Servings: 6 muffins Prep Time: 10 minutes Cook Time: 20 minutes Carbs per Serving: 5g

---

INGREDIENTS

- 6 large eggs
- 1 cup broccoli florets, finely chopped
- 1/2 cup shredded cheddar cheese
- 1/4 cup red bell pepper, diced
- Salt and pepper to taste

DIRECTIONS

1. Preheat the oven to 350°F (175°C) and grease a muffin tin.
2. In a bowl, whisk the eggs and season with salt and pepper.
3. Stir in the broccoli, cheese, and bell pepper.
4. Pour the mixture into the muffin tin and bake for 20 minutes or until set.

Nutrient Content (per serving):

- Calories: 150
- Total Fat: 10g
- Protein: 12g
- Carbohydrates: 5g
- Sugars: 2g
- Fiber: 1g
- Sodium: 180mg

"Healthy eating is a form of self-respect."

INGREDIENT TIPS:

- Broccoli is high in fiber and nutrients, making it excellent for blood sugar control.
- Eggs and cheese provide a good source of protein and calcium.

CINNAMON ALMOND PORRIDGE

A warm and comforting porridge with the sweet spice of cinnamon, ideal for a cozy breakfast.

Servings: 1 Prep Time: 5 minutes Cook Time: 10 minutes Carbs per Serving: 20g

---

INGREDIENTS

- 1/4 cup almond flour
- 1 cup unsweetened almond milk
- 1 tbsp ground flaxseed
- 1/2 tsp cinnamon
- Stevia to taste

DIRECTIONS

1. In a pot, combine almond flour, almond milk, flaxseed, and cinnamon.
2. Cook over medium heat, stirring constantly until it thickens.
3. Sweeten with stevia to taste and serve warm.

Nutrient Content (per serving):
- Calories: 200
- Total Fat: 15g
- Protein: 8g
- Carbohydrates: 20g
- Sugars: 1g
- Fiber: 5g
- Sodium: 100mg

"Wellness starts with the first bite."

INGREDIENT TIPS:
- Almond flour and flaxseed are low in carbs and high in healthy fats and fiber.
- Cinnamon may help lower blood sugar levels and improve insulin sensitivity.

SMOKED SALMON AND AVOCADO WRAP

A delicious and nutritious wrap that combines the richness of smoked salmon with creamy avocado, perfect for a savory breakfast or brunch.

Servings: 1 Prep Time: 5 minutes Cook Time: 0 minutes Carbs per Serving: 15g

---

INGREDIENTS

- 1 low-carb whole wheat wrap
- 2 oz smoked salmon
- 1/2 avocado, mashed
- 1 tbsp cream cheese
- 1/4 cup arugula
- Lemon juice to taste

DIRECTIONS

1. Spread the cream cheese over the wrap.
2. Top with mashed avocado, smoked salmon, and arugula.
3. Drizzle with lemon juice and roll up the wrap tightly.

Nutrient Content (per serving):

- Calories: 300
- Total Fat: 20g
- Protein: 15g
- Carbohydrates: 15g
- Sugars: 2g
- Fiber: 7g
- Sodium: 400mg

"Food is the most powerful medicine."

INGREDIENT TIPS:
- Smoked salmon is a great source of omega-3 fatty acids and protein.
- Avocado provides heart-healthy monounsaturated fats and fiber.

MEDITERRANEAN VEGGIE OMELETTE

A flavorful omelette that brings the tastes of the Mediterranean to your breakfast table, perfect for a nutritious start to the day.

Servings: 1 Prep Time: 5 minutes Cook Time: 10 minutes Carbs per Serving: 12g

INGREDIENTS

- 2 large eggs
- 1/4 cup spinach, chopped
- 2 tbsp red onion, diced
- 2 tbsp bell pepper, diced
- 1/4 cup cherry tomatoes, halved
- 1 tbsp crumbled feta cheese
- 1 tsp olive oil
- Salt and pepper to taste

DIRECTIONS

1. Beat the eggs in a bowl and season with salt and pepper.
2. Heat olive oil in a pan over medium heat.
3. Sauté onions and bell peppers until soft.
4. Add spinach and tomatoes, cook until spinach is wilted.
5. Pour the eggs over the veggies and let them set slightly.
6. Sprinkle feta cheese on top and fold the omelette in half.
7. Cook until the cheese is slightly melted and the eggs are cooked to your liking.

Nutrient Content (per serving):

- Calories: 250
- Total Fat: 18g
- Protein: 15g
- Carbohydrates: 12g
- Sugars: 6g
- Fiber: 3g
- Sodium: 320mg

"Take care of your body, it's the only place you have to live."

INGREDIENT TIPS:

- The Mediterranean diet is known for its health benefits, including blood sugar management1.
- Feta cheese adds flavor without too much fat, and the veggies provide fiber and nutrients.

PUMPKIN SEED AND ALMOND YOGURT

A simple yet satisfying yogurt dish sprinkled with crunchy seeds and nuts for a quick and healthy breakfast option.

Servings: 1 Prep Time: 5 minutes Cook Time: 0 minutes Carbs per Serving: 15g

---

INGREDIENTS

- 3/4 cup plain Greek yogurt
- 2 tbsp pumpkin seeds
- 1 tbsp sliced almonds
- 1/4 tsp vanilla extract
- Stevia to taste

DIRECTIONS

1. Mix the Greek yogurt with vanilla extract and sweeten with stevia.
2. Top with pumpkin seeds and sliced almonds.

Nutrient Content (per serving):

- Calories: 220
- Total Fat: 12g
- Protein: 20g
- Carbohydrates: 15g
- Sugars: 4g
- Fiber: 3g
- Sodium: 60mg

"Eat for the body you want, not for the body you have."

INGREDIENT TIPS:
- Greek yogurt is high in protein and can help keep blood sugar levels stable.
- Pumpkin seeds and almonds add healthy fats and magnesium, which is beneficial for blood sugar control.

AVOCADO AND EGG BREAKFAST SALAD

A fresh and hearty salad that combines creamy avocado with protein-rich eggs for a breakfast that's both nutritious and delicious.

Servings: 1 Prep Time: 10 minutes Cook Time: 5 minutes Carbs per Serving: 10g

INGREDIENTS

- 1 boiled egg, sliced
- 1/2 avocado, diced
- 1 cup mixed salad greens
- 1 tbsp olive oil
- 1 tsp lemon juice
- Salt and pepper to taste

DIRECTIONS

1. Arrange the salad greens on a plate.
2. Top with sliced boiled egg and diced avocado.
3. Drizzle with olive oil and lemon juice.
4. Season with salt and pepper to taste.

Nutrient Content (per serving):
- Calories: 300
- Total Fat: 25g
- Protein: 10g
- Carbohydrates: 10g
- Sugars: 2g
- Fiber: 7g
- Sodium: 200mg

"Health is the greatest gift."

INGREDIENT TIPS:
- Avocado is rich in monounsaturated fats and helps in maintaining healthy blood sugar levels.
- Eggs are a great source of protein and keep you feeling full longer.

Vegetarian Mains and Sides

Embracing a vegetarian diet can be a powerful way to manage pre-diabetes, offering a wealth of nutrients that support overall health and stabilize blood sugar levels. In this chapter, "Vegetarian Mains and Sides Recipes for Pre-Diabetic Diet," you'll find an array of flavorful and nutritious dishes tailored for those over 50 who are navigating pre-diabetes.

As we age, our dietary needs evolve, and it's important to focus on foods that are rich in fiber, vitamins, and minerals while being mindful of their impact on blood sugar. This chapter provides a collection of satisfying vegetarian main courses and sides that are both delicious and diabetes-friendly. From hearty legumes and whole grains to vibrant vegetables and plant-based proteins, these recipes will help you create balanced meals that are low in unhealthy fats and refined sugars.

Whether you're a lifelong vegetarian or exploring plant-based eating for the first time, these recipes are designed to be easy to prepare and packed with flavor. Enjoy dishes that not only nourish your body but also delight your taste buds, making it easier to maintain a healthy diet and lifestyle. Let's dive into the world of vegetarian cooking and discover meals that support your journey to better health and well-being.

QUINOA AND BLACK BEAN STUFFED PEPPERS

A colorful and nutritious dish that's as pleasing to the eye as it is to the palate, perfect for a hearty lunch or dinner.

Servings: 4 Prep Time: 15 minutes Cook Time: 30 minutes Carbs per Serving: 30g

INGREDIENTS

- 4 large bell peppers, halved and seeded
- 1 cup cooked quinoa
- 1 can black beans, drained and rinsed
- 1 cup corn kernels
- 1/2 cup diced tomatoes
- 1/4 cup chopped cilantro
- 1 tsp cumin
- Salt and pepper to taste
- 1/2 cup shredded low-fat cheese

DIRECTIONS

1. Preheat the oven to 375°F (190°C).
2. In a bowl, mix quinoa, black beans, corn, tomatoes, cilantro, cumin, salt, and pepper.
3. Stuff the bell pepper halves with the mixture and place in a baking dish.
4. Top with cheese and bake for 30 minutes until peppers are tender.

Nutrient Content (per serving):

- Calories: 250
- Total Fat: 5g
- Protein: 12g
- Carbohydrates: 30g
- Sugars: 5g
- Fiber: 9g
- Sodium: 200mg

"Your diet is a bank account. Good food choices are good investments."

INGREDIENT TIPS:

- Quinoa is a complete protein and has a low glycemic index, which is beneficial for blood sugar control.
- Black beans are high in fiber and protein, helping to prevent glucose spikes.

LENTIL AND MUSHROOM SHEPHERD'S PIE

A comforting and filling pie that brings a healthy twist to a classic dish, ideal for a satisfying meal that supports blood sugar management.

Servings: 6 Prep Time: 20 minutes Cook Time: 40 minutes Carbs per Serving: 35g

---

INGREDIENTS

- 2 cups brown lentils, cooked
- 1 cup mushrooms, chopped
- 1 onion, diced
- 2 cloves garlic, minced
- 1 cup frozen peas and carrots
- 2 tbsp tomato paste
- 1 tsp thyme
- Salt and pepper to taste
- 2 cups mashed sweet potatoes

DIRECTIONS

1. Sauté onions, garlic, and mushrooms until soft.
2. Add lentils, peas, carrots, tomato paste, thyme, salt, and pepper. Cook for 10 minutes.
3. Transfer to a baking dish and top with mashed sweet potatoes.
4. Bake at 375°F (190°C) for 30 minutes until the top is golden.

Nutrient Content (per serving):
- Calories: 300
- Total Fat: 2g
- Protein: 14g
- Carbohydrates: 35g
- Sugars: 7g
- Fiber: 11g
- Sodium: 250mg

"Eat clean, feel great."

INGREDIENT TIPS:
- Lentils are a great source of plant-based protein and fiber, which can help stabilize blood sugar levels.
- Sweet potatoes have a lower glycemic index than white potatoes and provide a sweet taste without a significant sugar spike.

ROASTED CAULIFLOWER AND CHICKPEA CURRY

A flavorful curry that's both warming and nutritious, perfect for those looking to enjoy a rich, creamy dish without worrying about blood sugar spikes.

Servings: 4 Prep Time: 15 minutes Cook Time: 30 minutes Carbs per Serving: 25g

---

INGREDIENTS

- 1 head cauliflower, cut into florets
- 1 can chickpeas, drained and rinsed
- 1 can coconut milk
- 1 tbsp curry powder
- 1 tsp turmeric
- Salt to taste
- Fresh cilantro for garnish

DIRECTIONS

1. Roast cauliflower florets at 400°F (200°C) for 20 minutes until slightly crispy.
2. In a pot, combine chickpeas, coconut milk, curry powder, turmeric, and salt. Simmer for 10 minutes.
3. Add roasted cauliflower to the pot and cook for another 5 minutes.
4. Garnish with cilantro before serving.

Nutrient Content (per serving):
- Calories: 280
- Total Fat: 14g
- Protein: 10g
- Carbohydrates: 25g
- Sugars: 5g
- Fiber: 9g
- Sodium: 300mg

"Nourish to flourish."

INGREDIENT TIPS:
- Cauliflower is a non-starchy vegetable that's low in carbs and high in fiber.
- Chickpeas are a good source of protein and have a low glycemic index, making them excellent for blood sugar control.

ZUCCHINI NOODLES WITH PESTO AND CHERRY TOMATOES

A light and fresh dish that's quick to prepare, offering a burst of flavor with every bite while being kind to your blood sugar levels.

Servings: 2 Prep Time: 10 minutes Cook Time: 5 minutes Carbs per Serving: 15g

---

INGREDIENTS

- 2 large zucchinis, spiralized
- 1 cup cherry tomatoes, halved
- 1/4 cup pesto sauce
- Salt and pepper to taste
- Grated Parmesan cheese for garnish

DIRECTIONS

1. Sauté zucchini noodles in a pan for 2-3 minutes until tender.
2. Add cherry tomatoes and pesto sauce, cook for another 2 minutes.
3. Season with salt and pepper.
4. Serve with a sprinkle of Parmesan cheese.

Nutrient Content (per serving):
- Calories: 180
- Total Fat: 12g
- Protein: 6g
- Carbohydrates: 15g
- Sugars: 8g
- Fiber: 4g
- Sodium: 250mg

"Eating healthy is a form of self-love."

INGREDIENT TIPS:
- Zucchini noodles are a low-carb alternative to pasta and can help reduce blood sugar levels after meals.
- Cherry tomatoes add freshness and are low on the glycemic index.

EGGPLANT AND TOFU STIR-FRY

A hearty stir-fry that's full of flavor and texture, making it a satisfying main course that supports a healthy blood sugar level.

Servings: 4 Prep Time: 15 minutes Cook Time: 15 minutes Carbs per Serving: 20g

INGREDIENTS

- 1 large eggplant, cubed
- 1 block firm tofu, drained and cubed
- 1 bell pepper, sliced
- 2 tbsp soy sauce
- 1 tbsp sesame oil
- 1 tsp ginger, minced
- 1 clove garlic, minced
- Green onions for garnish

DIRECTIONS

1. Heat sesame oil in a pan and sauté garlic and ginger until fragrant.
2. Add eggplant and bell pepper, cook until tender.
3. Add tofu and soy sauce, stir-fry for 5 minutes.
4. Garnish with green onions before serving.

Nutrient Content (per serving):
- Calories: 200
- Total Fat: 10g
- Protein: 12g
- Carbohydrates: 20g
- Sugars: 8g
- Fiber: 6g
- Sodium: 400mg

"Your health is an investment, not an expense."

INGREDIENT TIPS:
- Eggplant is a fiber-rich vegetable that can help in blood sugar management.
- Tofu is a low-fat source of protein that doesn't affect blood sugar levels significantly.

BALSAMIC ROASTED BRUSSELS SPROUTS

A simple yet flavorful side dish that pairs well with any main course, offering a delightful mix of textures and tastes.

Servings: 4 Prep Time: 10 minutes Cook Time: 25 minutes Carbs per Serving: 15g

---

INGREDIENTS

- 1 lb Brussels sprouts, halved
- 2 tbsp olive oil
- 2 tbsp balsamic vinegar
- Salt and pepper to taste
- 1 tbsp chopped walnuts (optional)

DIRECTIONS

1. Preheat the oven to 400°F (200°C).
2. Toss Brussels sprouts with olive oil, balsamic vinegar, salt, and pepper.
3. Spread on a baking sheet and roast for 25 minutes until caramelized.
4. Top with chopped walnuts for added crunch before serving.

Nutrient Content (per serving):
- Calories: 120
- Total Fat: 7g
- Protein: 4g
- Carbohydrates: 15g
- Sugars: 3g
- Fiber: 4g
- Sodium: 30mg

"A healthy outside starts from the inside."

INGREDIENT TIPS:
- Brussels sprouts are high in fiber and nutrients, which can help regulate blood sugar levels.
- Balsamic vinegar adds flavor without significantly increasing sugar content.

STUFFED ACORN SQUASH WITH QUINOA AND CRANBERRIES

A festive and hearty dish that's perfect for a special occasion or a cozy night in, filled with the goodness of whole grains and autumn flavors.

Servings: 4 Prep Time: 15 minutes Cook Time: 40 minutes Carbs per Serving: 30g

INGREDIENTS

- 2 acorn squashes, halved and seeded
- 1 cup cooked quinoa
- 1/4 cup dried cranberries
- 1/4 cup chopped pecans
- 1/4 tsp cinnamon
- Salt to taste
- 1 tbsp maple syrup (optional)

DIRECTIONS

1. Preheat the oven to 375°F (190°C).
2. Place acorn squash halves cut-side down on a baking sheet and bake for 20 minutes.
3. In a bowl, mix quinoa, cranberries, pecans, cinnamon, and salt.
4. Turn squash halves cut-side up and fill with the quinoa mixture.
5. Drizzle with maple syrup if desired and bake for another 20 minutes.

Nutrient Content (per serving):
- Calories: 250
- Total Fat: 8g
- Protein: 5g
- Carbohydrates: 30g
- Sugars: 10g
- Fiber: 5g
- Sodium: 20mg

"Savor the flavor of healthy living."

INGREDIENT TIPS:
- Acorn squash is a good source of complex carbohydrates and fiber.
- Quinoa provides complete protein and helps keep blood sugar levels stable.

LEMON GARLIC ROASTED ASPARAGUS

A light and zesty side dish that's quick to prepare and adds a burst of flavor to any meal, while being friendly to your blood sugar levels.

Servings: 4 Prep Time: 5 minutes Cook Time: 15 minutes Carbs per Serving: 5g

---

INGREDIENTS

- 1 lb asparagus, trimmed
- 2 tbsp olive oil
- 2 cloves garlic, minced
- 1 lemon, juice and zest
- Salt and pepper to taste

DIRECTIONS

1. Preheat the oven to 425°F (220°C).
2. Toss asparagus with olive oil, garlic, lemon juice, zest, salt, and pepper.
3. Spread on a baking sheet and roast for 15 minutes until tender.

Nutrient Content (per serving):
- Calories: 80
- Total Fat: 7g
- Protein: 2g
- Carbohydrates: 5g
- Sugars: 2g
- Fiber: 2g
- Sodium: 2mg

"Eating well is a form of self-respect."

INGREDIENT TIPS:
- Asparagus is low in carbohydrates and high in fiber, making it an excellent choice for blood sugar management.
- Lemon adds a refreshing flavor without adding sugar.

BARLEY AND ROASTED VEGETABLE PILAF

A hearty and rustic pilaf that combines the chewiness of barley with the sweetness of roasted vegetables, perfect for a satisfying main or side dish.

Servings: 4 Prep Time: 15 minutes Cook Time: 40 minutes Carbs per Serving: 35g

INGREDIENTS

- 1 cup pearl barley
- 2 cups vegetable broth
- 1 zucchini, diced
- 1 red bell pepper, diced
- 1 yellow squash, diced
- 1 red onion, diced
- 2 tbsp olive oil
- Salt and pepper to taste
- Fresh parsley, chopped (for garnish)

DIRECTIONS

1. Preheat the oven to 400°F (200°C).
2. Toss zucchini, bell pepper, squash, and onion with olive oil, salt, and pepper.
3. Roast vegetables for 20 minutes until tender and slightly caramelized.
4. Meanwhile, bring vegetable broth to a boil, add barley, and simmer covered for 30 minutes.
5. Combine cooked barley with roasted vegetables.
6. Garnish with fresh parsley before serving.

Nutrient Content (per serving):
- Calories: 300
- Total Fat: 7g
- Protein: 8g
- Carbohydrates: 35g
- Sugars: 5g
- Fiber: 9g
- Sodium: 150mg

"Healthy eating is a lifestyle, not a diet."

INGREDIENT TIPS:
- Barley is a whole grain that's high in fiber and has a low glycemic index, which can help manage blood sugar levels.
- Roasted vegetables add flavor and antioxidants without significantly impacting blood sugar.

SPAGHETTI SQUASH PRIMAVERA

A light and colorful dish that's as nutritious as it is delicious, offering a pasta-like experience without the worry of raising blood sugar levels.

Servings: 4 Prep Time: 10 minutes Cook Time: 45 minutes Carbs per Serving: 20g

---

INGREDIENTS

- 1 large spaghetti squash
- 1 cup cherry tomatoes, halved
- 1 cup broccoli florets
- 1/2 cup sliced carrots
- 1/4 cup peas
- 2 cloves garlic, minced
- 2 tbsp olive oil
- Salt and pepper to taste
- Grated Parmesan cheese (optional)

DIRECTIONS

1. Cut spaghetti squash in half lengthwise and remove seeds.
2. Place cut-side down on a baking sheet and bake at 375°F (190°C) for 35 minutes.
3. Sauté garlic, tomatoes, broccoli, carrots, and peas in olive oil until tender.
4. Use a fork to scrape the squash into strands and mix with the sautéed vegetables.
5. Season with salt and pepper, and top with Parmesan cheese if desired.

Nutrient Content (per serving):
- Calories: 180
- Total Fat: 7g
- Protein: 4g
- Carbohydrates: 20g
- Sugars: 7g
- Fiber: 4g
- Sodium: 100mg

"Balance, variety, and moderation lead to health and happiness."

INGREDIENT TIPS:
- Spaghetti squash is a low-carb alternative to pasta and helps prevent blood sugar spikes.
- A variety of vegetables increases nutrient intake and fiber, which is beneficial for blood sugar control.

CHICKPEA AND SPINACH CURRY

A comforting curry that's bursting with flavor and packed with nutrients, making it an ideal meal for those managing blood sugar levels.

Servings: 4 Prep Time: 10 minutes Cook Time: 20 minutes Carbs per Serving: 30g

---

INGREDIENTS

- 1 can chickpeas, drained and rinsed
- 2 cups fresh spinach
- 1 onion, diced
- 2 cloves garlic, minced
- 1 tbsp curry powder
- 1 tsp cumin
- 1 can diced tomatoes
- 1 can coconut milk
- Salt to taste
- Fresh cilantro for garnish

DIRECTIONS

1. Sauté onion and garlic until translucent.
2. Add curry powder and cumin, cook for 1 minute.
3. Stir in chickpeas, tomatoes, and coconut milk. Simmer for 15 minutes.
4. Add spinach and cook until wilted.
5. Season with salt and garnish with cilantro before serving.

Nutrient Content (per serving):
- Calories: 280
- Total Fat: 12g
- Protein: 10g
- Carbohydrates: 30g
- Sugars: 6g
- Fiber: 8g
- Sodium: 300mg

"Health is the greatest gift."

INGREDIENT TIPS:
- Chickpeas are a great source of protein and fiber, which can help stabilize blood sugar levels.
- Spinach is low in carbs and high in vitamins and minerals, supporting overall health.

Chapter Five

Soup and Stew

Warm, comforting, and incredibly nutritious, soups and stews are perfect for those managing pre-diabetes, especially for individuals over 50. In this chapter, "Soup and Stew Recipes for Pre-Diabetic Diet," you'll discover a variety of delicious recipes designed to help you maintain stable blood sugar levels while enjoying satisfying, hearty meals.

Soups and stews are ideal for incorporating a wide range of vegetables, lean proteins, and whole grains into your diet, providing a nutrient-dense option that is both filling and flavorful. These recipes focus on using ingredients that are low in glycemic index and high in fiber, ensuring that your meals support healthy blood sugar levels.

From classic vegetable soups to protein-rich stews and everything in between, this chapter offers something for every palate. These dishes are not only easy to prepare but also perfect for batch cooking, allowing you to enjoy healthy meals throughout the week with minimal effort.

Dive into this collection of wholesome soups and stews and discover how these comforting dishes can be a delicious part of your pre-diabetic diet. Embrace the warmth and nourishment they provide as you take steps toward a healthier, more balanced lifestyle.

LENTIL VEGETABLE SOUP

A hearty and nutritious soup that's perfect for a cold day, packed with fiber-rich vegetables and lentils to keep blood sugar levels steady.

Servings: 4 Prep Time: 10 minutes Cook Time: 30 minutes Carbs per Serving: 20g

---

INGREDIENTS

- 1 cup dried lentils, rinsed
- 4 cups low-sodium vegetable broth
- 1 cup diced carrots
- 1 cup diced celery
- 1 cup chopped spinach
- 1/2 cup diced onions
- 2 cloves garlic, minced
- 1 tsp olive oil
- 1 tsp turmeric
- Salt and pepper to taste

Nutrient Content (per serving):
- Calories: 240
- Total Fat: 3g
- Protein: 14g
- Carbohydrates: 20g
- Sugars: 3g
- Fiber: 8g
- Sodium: 120mg

DIRECTIONS

1. Heat olive oil in a large pot over medium heat.
2. Sauté onions and garlic until translucent.
3. Add carrots and celery, cook for 5 minutes.
4. Pour in vegetable broth and lentils. Bring to a boil.
5. Reduce heat, add turmeric, and simmer for 20 minutes.
6. Stir in spinach and cook until wilted.
7. Season with salt and pepper to taste.

"Healthy food fuels a healthy life."

INGREDIENT TIPS:
- Lentils are a low-glycemic index food, rich in fiber and protein, which can help manage blood sugar level.
- Turmeric has anti-inflammatory properties and may aid in blood sugar control.

TOMATO AND WHITE BEAN STEW

A comforting stew that combines the robust flavors of tomatoes and herbs with the creaminess of white beans, offering a filling meal that supports blood sugar management.

Servings: 4   Prep Time: 10 minutes   Cook Time: 25 minutes   Carbs per Serving: 25g

---

INGREDIENTS

- 1 can white beans, drained and rinsed
- 2 cups diced tomatoes
- 1 cup chopped kale
- 1/2 cup diced bell peppers
- 1/2 cup diced zucchini
- 1 quart low-sodium vegetable broth
- 1 tsp dried basil
- 1 tsp dried oregano
- Salt and pepper to taste

DIRECTIONS

1. In a large pot, bring vegetable broth to a simmer.
2. Add tomatoes, bell peppers, zucchini, basil, and oregano.
3. Cook for 15 minutes until vegetables are tender.
4. Stir in white beans and kale, cook for an additional 10 minutes.
5. Season with salt and pepper.

Nutrient Content (per serving):
- Calories: 200
- Total Fat: 1g
- Protein: 10g
- Carbohydrates: 25g
- Sugars: 4g
- Fiber: 6g
- Sodium: 150mg

"Every healthy choice brings you closer to a better you."

INGREDIENT TIPS:
- White beans have a low glycemic index and are a good source of protein and fiber1.
- Kale is nutrient-dense and may help in managing blood sugar levels1.

CHICKEN AND BARLEY SOUP

A wholesome soup that's both warming and satisfying, featuring lean protein from chicken and fiber from barley to help maintain stable blood sugar levels.

Servings: 4   Prep Time: 15 minutes   Cook Time: 40 minutes   Carbs per Serving: 30g

INGREDIENTS

- 1/2 lb chicken breast, cubed
- 1/2 cup pearl barley
- 4 cups low-sodium chicken broth
- 1 cup diced butternut squash
- 1 cup chopped leeks
- 1/2 cup sliced mushrooms
- 1 tsp thyme
- Salt and pepper to taste
-

DIRECTIONS

1. In a large pot, brown chicken cubes over medium heat.
2. Add leeks and mushrooms, cook until softened.
3. Pour in chicken broth and bring to a boil.
4. Add barley, butternut squash, and thyme.
5. Reduce heat to a simmer and cook for 30 minutes.
6. Season with salt and pepper to taste.

Nutrient Content (per serving):
- Calories: 260
- Total Fat: 3g
- Protein: 20g
- Carbohydrates: 30g
- Sugars: 3g
- Fiber: 6g
- Sodium: 200mg

"Let food be thy medicine and medicine be thy food."

INGREDIENT TIPS:
- Barley is a whole grain with a low glycemic index, contributing to a slower rise in blood sugar levels.
- Butternut squash provides complex carbohydrates and fiber.

AUTUMN BISQUE

An autumn-inspired bisque that warms the soul, combining the earthy flavors of rutabaga and leeks with a touch of thyme. Perfect for cozy evenings!

Servings: 6   Prep Time: 15 minutes   Cook Time: 40 minutes   Carbs per Serving: 25g

---

INGREDIENTS

- 1 medium rutabaga, peeled and cubed
- 2 leeks, white and light green parts, sliced
- 2 cloves garlic, minced
- 1 tbsp olive oil
- 4 cups low-sodium vegetable broth
- 1 cup unsweetened almond milk
- 1 tsp dried thyme
- Salt and pepper to taste
- Fresh parsley for garnish

Nutrient Content (per serving):
- Calories: 150
- Total Fat: 5g
- Protein: 3g
- Carbohydrates: 25g
- Sugars: 8g
- Fiber: 6g
- Sodium: 200mg

DIRECTIONS

1. In a large pot, sauté leeks and garlic in olive oil until softened.
2. Add rutabaga cubes, vegetable broth, and thyme. Bring to a boil.
3. Reduce heat and simmer for 30 minutes until rutabaga is tender.
4. Use an immersion blender to puree the soup until smooth.
5. Stir in almond milk and season with salt and pepper.
6. Garnish with fresh parsley before serving.

"Your health journey starts with a single step."

INGREDIENT TIPS:
- Rutabaga is a low-carb root vegetable that adds natural sweetness and creaminess to the soup.
- Leeks provide flavor without significantly affecting blood sugar levels.

GREENS AND BEANS TURKEY SOUP

A comforting and hearty soup that combines tender turkey, nutrient-rich kale, and creamy kidney beans. Perfect for using up leftover holiday turkey!

Servings: 6   Prep Time: 10 minutes   Cook Time: 1 hour   Carbs per Serving: 20g

---

INGREDIENTS

- 1 lb cooked turkey (from leftover roasted turkey or store-bought)
- 1 cup chopped kale
- 1 cup canned kidney beans, drained and rinsed
- 1 cup diced carrots
- 1 cup diced celery
- 1 onion, chopped
- 2 cloves garlic, minced
- 4 cups low-sodium chicken broth
- 1 tsp dried thyme
- Salt and pepper to taste

Nutrient Content (per serving):
- Calories: 180
- Total Fat: 3g
- Protein: 20g
- Carbohydrates: 20g
- Sugars: 4g
- Fiber: 6g
- Sodium: 150mg

DIRECTIONS

1. In a large pot, sauté onions and garlic until translucent.
2. Add carrots, celery, and thyme. Cook for 5 minutes.
3. Pour in chicken broth and bring to a boil.
4. Add cooked turkey, kale, and kidney beans. Simmer for 30 minutes.
5. Season with salt and pepper.

"Eat right, be bright."

INGREDIENT TIPS:

- Kale is a nutrient powerhouse and adds vitamins and minerals to the soup.
- Kidney beans provide protein and fiber, helping stabilize blood sugar levels.

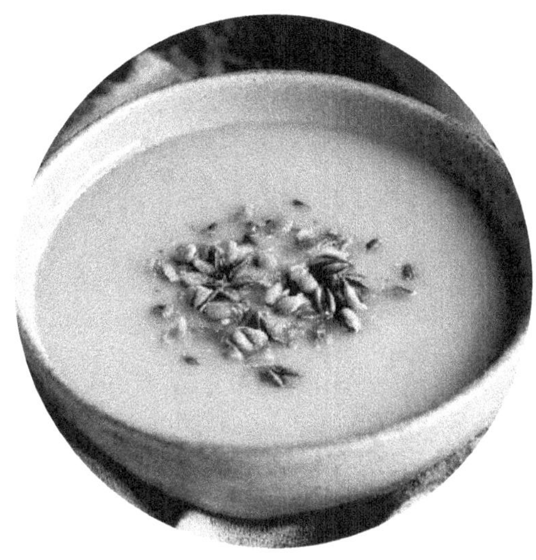

BUTTERNUT SQUASH AND APPLE SOUP

A velvety and comforting butternut squash soup with a hint of sweetness from apples and warming spices, offering a delicious and nourishing meal option.

Servings: 4 | Prep Time: 15 mins | Cook Time: 45 mins | Carbs per Serving: 30g

INGREDIENTS

- 1 butternut squash, peeled, seeded, and cubed
- 2 apples, peeled, cored, and chopped
- 1 onion, chopped
- 2 cloves garlic, minced
- 4 cups vegetable broth
- 1 teaspoon ground cinnamon
- 1/2 teaspoon ground nutmeg
- Salt and pepper to taste
- 2 tablespoons olive oil
- Greek yogurt for garnish (optional)
- Toasted pumpkin seeds for garnish (optional)

DIRECTIONS

1. Preheat the oven to 400°F (200°C).
2. Place butternut squash cubes and chopped apples on a baking sheet.
3. Drizzle with olive oil, sprinkle with salt, pepper, cinnamon, and nutmeg. Toss to coat.
4. Roast in the oven for 25-30 minutes until tender and caramelized.
5. In a large pot, heat olive oil over medium heat.
6. Add onions and garlic, sauté until softened.
7. Add roasted butternut squash, apples, and vegetable broth.
8. Bring to a boil, then reduce heat and simmer for 10-15 minutes.
9. Use an immersion blender to blend the soup until smooth.
10. Season with salt and pepper to taste.
11. Serve hot, garnished with a dollop of Greek yogurt and toasted pumpkin seeds if desired.

NUTRIENT CONTENT (PER SERVING):		INGREDIENT TIPS:
• Calories: 220	• Sugars: 10g	Butternut squash and apples provide natural sweetness. Greek yogurt adds creaminess and protein.
• Total Fat: 8g	• Fiber: 6g	
• Protein: 4g	• Sodium: 700mg	
• Carbohydrates: 30g		

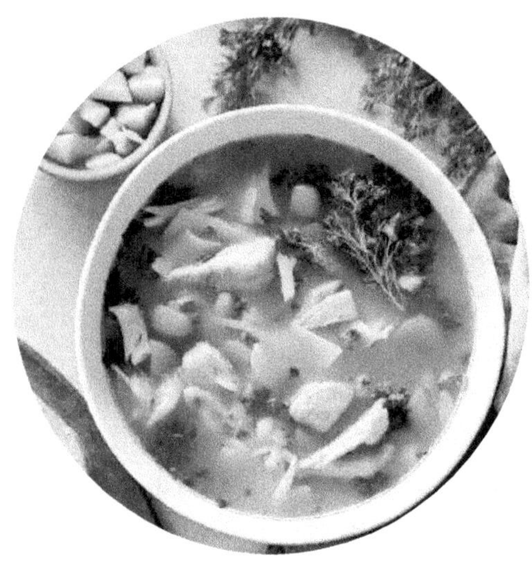

CHICKEN AND VEGETABLE SOUP

A comforting and nourishing chicken soup packed with vegetables and aromatic herbs, making it a satisfying meal option.

Servings: 6 | Prep Time: 15 mins | Cook Time: 25 mins | Carbs per Serving: 15g

INGREDIENTS

- 1 tablespoon olive oil
- 1 onion, chopped
- 2 carrots, diced
- 2 celery stalks, chopped
- 2 cloves garlic, minced
- 4 cups chicken broth
- 2 cups shredded cooked chicken
- 1 cup diced potatoes
- 1 cup chopped green beans
- 1 teaspoon dried thyme
- Salt and pepper to taste
- Fresh parsley for garnish

DIRECTIONS

1. In a large pot, heat olive oil over medium heat.
2. Add onions, carrots, celery, and garlic. Sauté until vegetables are tender.
3. Pour in chicken broth and bring to a boil.
4. Add shredded chicken, diced potatoes, chopped green beans, dried thyme, salt, and pepper.
5. Reduce heat and simmer for 20-25 minutes until vegetables are cooked through.
6. Adjust seasoning if needed.
7. Serve hot, garnished with fresh parsley.

"Small steps lead to big changes."

NUTRIENT CONTENT (PER SERVING):		INGREDIENT TIPS:
• Calories: 220 • Total Fat: 8g • Protein: 20g • Carbohydrates: 15g	• Sugars: 4g • Fiber: 3g • Sodium: 700mg	Chicken provides protein. Vegetables offer vitamins and fiber.

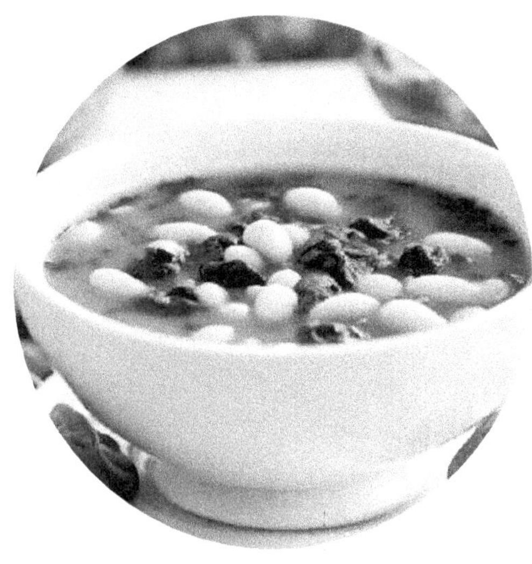

SPINACH AND WHITE BEAN SOUP

A wholesome and flavorful soup featuring white beans, spinach, and aromatic spices, offering a nutritious and delicious meal choice.

Servings: 6 | Prep Time: 10 mins | Cook Time: 20 mins | Carbs per Serving: 30g

INGREDIENTS

- 1 tablespoon olive oil
- 1 onion, chopped
- 2 cloves garlic, minced
- 4 cups vegetable broth
- 2 cans white beans, drained and rinsed
- 4 cups chopped fresh spinach
- 1 teaspoon dried rosemary
- 1 teaspoon paprika
- Salt and pepper to taste
- Lemon wedges for serving (optional)

DIRECTIONS

1. In a large pot, heat olive oil over medium heat.
2. Add onions and garlic, sauté until onions are translucent.
3. Pour in vegetable broth and bring to a simmer.
4. Add white beans, chopped spinach, dried rosemary, paprika, salt, and pepper.
5. Simmer for 15-20 minutes until flavors meld and spinach wilts.
6. Adjust seasoning if needed.
7. Serve hot with a squeeze of lemon juice if desired.

"You don't have to be perfect, just better than yesterday."

NUTRIENT CONTENT (PER SERVING):		INGREDIENT TIPS:
• Calories: 250 • Total Fat: 6g • Protein: 12g • Carbohydrates: 30g	• Sugars: 4g • Fiber: 7g • Sodium: 800mg	White beans provide protein and fiber. Spinach adds nutrients and greens.

Chapter Six

Meatless Main Dishes

Adopting a meatless diet can be a powerful strategy for managing pre-diabetes, offering a variety of health benefits while supporting stable blood sugar levels. In this chapter, "Meatless Main Dishes Recipes for Pre-Diabetic Diet," you'll find an inspiring collection of flavorful, nutrient-dense meals designed specifically for individuals over 50 navigating pre-diabetes.

As we age, it's essential to focus on foods that provide essential nutrients without spiking blood sugar levels. The meatless main dishes in this chapter highlight plant-based proteins, whole grains, and an abundance of vegetables, ensuring that each meal is balanced, satisfying, and diabetes-friendly. These recipes are crafted to deliver the right mix of fiber, vitamins, and minerals to support overall health and well-being.

From hearty grain bowls and bean-based dishes to creative vegetable entrees, this chapter offers a diverse range of options that prove you don't need meat to create delicious, fulfilling meals. Whether you're a seasoned vegetarian or just exploring plant-based eating, these recipes will help you enjoy the benefits of a meatless diet while keeping your blood sugar in check.

Get ready to discover a world of meatless culinary delights that are as nutritious as they are tasty. Embrace these dishes as part of your journey to better health and enjoy the rich flavors and variety they bring to your pre-diabetic diet.

ZUCCHINI NOODLES WITH PESTO

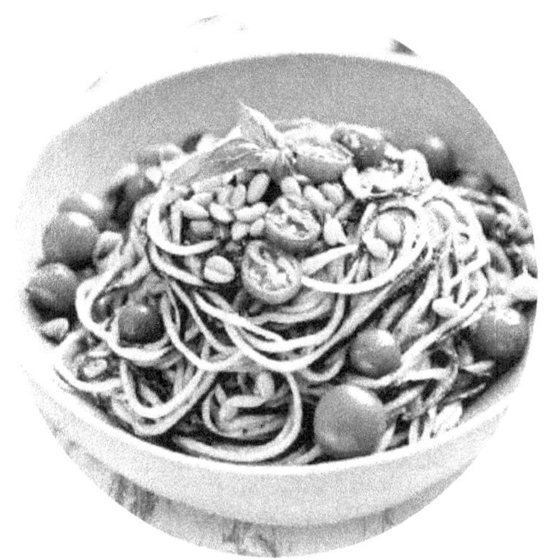

Light and refreshing zucchini noodles tossed in vibrant basil pesto with cherry tomatoes and pine nuts, a satisfying and low-carb meal choice.

Servings: 4 | Prep Time: 15 mins | Cook Time: 5 mins | Carbs per Serving: 10g

INGREDIENTS

- 4 medium zucchinis, spiralized into noodles
- 1 cup cherry tomatoes, halved
- 1/2 cup basil pesto (store-bought or homemade)
- 1/4 cup pine nuts, toasted
- 2 tablespoons olive oil
- 2 cloves garlic, minced
- Salt and pepper to taste
- Grated Parmesan cheese (optional for topping)

DIRECTIONS

1. Heat olive oil in a large skillet over medium heat.
2. Add minced garlic and sauté until fragrant.
3. Add spiralized zucchini noodles to the skillet and toss with the garlic oil.
4. Cook for 2-3 minutes until the noodles are just tender.
5. Stir in cherry tomatoes and cook for another minute.
6. Remove from heat and transfer the zucchini noodles and tomatoes to a serving dish.
7. Add basil pesto to the noodles and toss until evenly coated.
8. Sprinkle toasted pine nuts on top.
9. Season with salt and pepper to taste.
10. If desired, sprinkle grated Parmesan cheese over the noodles before serving.

NUTRIENT CONTENT (PER SERVING):		INGREDIENT TIPS:
• Calories: 220 • Total Fat: 18g • Protein: 4g • Carbohydrates: 10g	• Sugars: 5g • Fiber: 3g • Sodium: 120mg	Zucchini noodles are a low-carb alternative to pasta. Choose a low-sodium pesto for a healthier option.

LENTIL AND VEGETABLE STIR-FRY

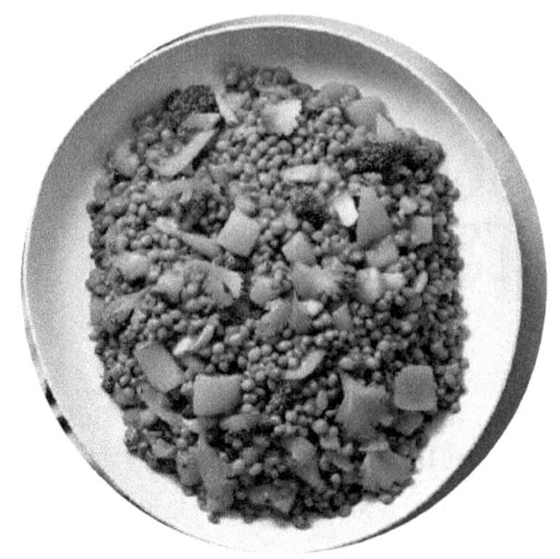

This quick and easy lentil and vegetable stir-fry is a perfect weeknight meal, packed with fiber and protein to help manage blood sugar levels.

Servings: 4 | Prep Time: 15 minutes | Cook Time: 30 minutes | Carbs per Serving: 35g

INGREDIENTS

- 1 cup lentils, rinsed and drained
- 2 cups water
- 1 tbsp olive oil
- 1 red bell pepper, sliced
- 1 yellow bell pepper, sliced
- 1 zucchini, sliced
- 1 cup broccoli florets
- 1 carrot, julienned
- 2 cloves garlic, minced
- 1 tbsp soy sauce (low sodium)
- 1 tsp sesame oil
- 1 tbsp chopped fresh ginger
- 1/4 cup chopped green onions
- 1 tbsp sesame seeds

DIRECTIONS

1. In a medium pot, combine lentils and water. Bring to a boil, reduce heat, and simmer for 20-25 minutes until tender. Drain and set aside.
2. Heat olive oil in a large skillet over medium-high heat. Add garlic and ginger, sauté for 1 minute.
3. Add all vegetables to the skillet and stir-fry for 5-7 minutes, until tender but still crisp.
4. Stir in cooked lentils, soy sauce, and sesame oil. Cook for an additional 2-3 minutes.
5. Garnish with green onions and sesame seeds. Serve immediately.

NUTRIENT CONTENT (PER SERVING):		INGREDIENT TIPS:
• Calories: 250 • Total Fat: 8g • Protein: 12g • Carbohydrates: 35g	• Sugars: 8g • Fiber: 12g • Sodium: 320mg	• Lentils: High in fiber and protein, with a low glycemic index, they help maintain blood sugar levels. • Vegetables: Non-starchy and full of fiber, aiding in digestion and glucose control.

CHICKPEA AND SPINACH CURRY

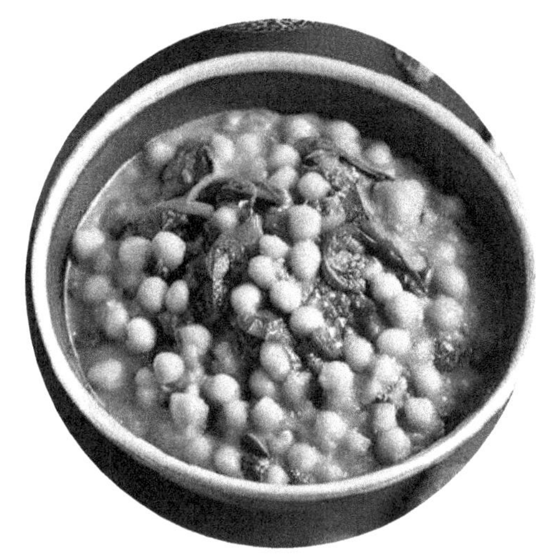

This creamy chickpea and spinach curry is rich in plant-based protein and fiber, providing a satisfying meal that helps manage blood sugar levels.

Servings: 4 | Prep Time: 10 minutes | Cook Time: 25 minutes | Carbs per Serving: 25g

INGREDIENTS

- 1 can (15 oz) chickpeas, drained and rinsed
- 2 cups fresh spinach, chopped
- 1 can (14 oz) diced tomatoes
- 1 small onion, chopped
- 2 cloves garlic, minced
- 1 tbsp ginger, minced
- 1 can (14 oz) light coconut milk
- 1 tbsp curry powder
- 1 tsp ground cumin
- 1 tsp turmeric
- 1 tbsp olive oil
- Salt and pepper to taste
- 1/4 cup fresh cilantro, chopped

DIRECTIONS

1. Heat olive oil in a large pot over medium heat. Add onion, garlic, and ginger, sauté until onion is translucent.
2. Stir in curry powder, cumin, and turmeric, and cook for 1 minute.
3. Add diced tomatoes and coconut milk, bring to a simmer.
4. Stir in chickpeas and spinach, and cook for 10-15 minutes until spinach is wilted and chickpeas are heated through.
5. Season with salt and pepper to taste. Garnish with fresh cilantro.
6. Serve hot.

NUTRIENT CONTENT (PER SERVING):	INGREDIENT TIPS:
• Calories: 280 • Total Fat: 14g • Protein: 9g • Carbohydrates: 25g • Sugars: 7g • Fiber: 7g • Sodium: 420mg	• Chickpeas: Low glycemic index and high in fiber, they help regulate blood sugar levels. • Spinach: Non-starchy vegetable, rich in nutrients and fiber.

EGGPLANT AND TOMATO STEW

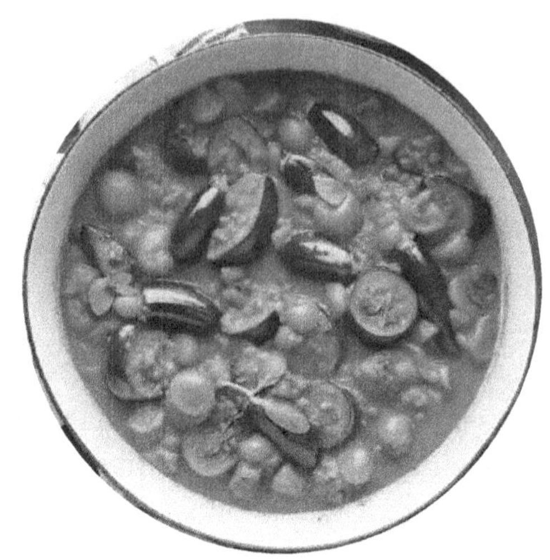

This hearty eggplant and tomato stew is packed with Mediterranean flavors and is ideal for a filling, diabetes-friendly meal.

Servings: 4 | Prep Time: 15 minutes | Cook Time: 30 minutes | Carbs per Serving: 22g

INGREDIENTS

- 2 large eggplants, diced
- 2 cups cherry tomatoes, halved
- 1 onion, chopped
- 3 cloves garlic, minced
- 1 can (15 oz) chickpeas, drained and rinsed
- 2 tbsp olive oil
- 1 tsp dried oregano
- 1 tsp dried basil
- 1/2 tsp black pepper
- 1/2 tsp salt
- 1/4 cup fresh parsley, chopped

DIRECTIONS

1. Heat olive oil in a large pot over medium heat. Add onion and garlic, sauté until softened.
2. Add eggplant and cook until it begins to soften, about 5 minutes.
3. Stir in tomatoes, chickpeas, oregano, basil, salt, and pepper. Simmer for 20-25 minutes, until vegetables are tender.
4. Garnish with fresh parsley and serve warm.

NUTRIENT CONTENT (PER SERVING):

- Calories: 220
- Total Fat: 10g
- Protein: 6g
- Carbohydrates: 22g
- Sugars: 8g
- Fiber: 9g
- Sodium: 380mg

INGREDIENT TIPS:

- Eggplant: Low in carbohydrates and high in fiber, which helps manage blood sugar.
- Tomatoes: Non-starchy vegetable that adds flavor and nutrients.
- Chickpeas: Provide protein and fiber, helping to stabilize glucose levels.

CAULIFLOWER AND CHICKPEA TACOS

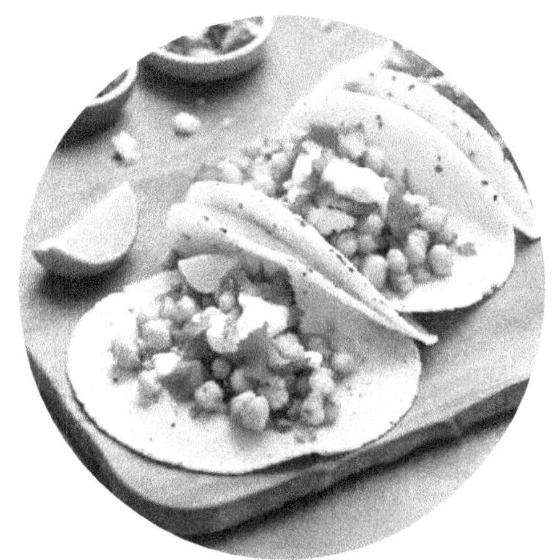

These vibrant cauliflower and chickpea tacos are a delicious, diabetes-friendly alternative to traditional tacos, packed with fiber and flavor.

Servings: 4 | Prep Time: 15 minutes | Cook Time: 30 minutes | Carbs per Serving: 22g

INGREDIENTS

- 1 head cauliflower, cut into florets
- 1 can (15 oz) chickpeas, drained and rinsed
- 2 tbsp olive oil
- 1 tbsp chili powder
- 1 tsp cumin
- 1 tsp paprika
- 1/2 tsp garlic powder
- 1/2 tsp salt
- 1/4 tsp black pepper
- 8 small whole wheat tortillas
- 1 cup shredded lettuce
- 1/2 cup diced tomatoes
- 1/4 cup chopped fresh cilantro
- 1/4 cup plain Greek yogurt (optional)

DIRECTIONS

1. Preheat oven to 400°F (200°C).
2. In a large bowl, toss cauliflower florets and chickpeas with olive oil, chili powder, cumin, paprika, garlic powder, salt, and black pepper.
3. Spread mixture on a baking sheet and roast for 25-30 minutes, until cauliflower is tender and chickpeas are crispy.
4. Warm tortillas according to package instructions.
5. Assemble tacos by placing roasted cauliflower and chickpeas on tortillas.
6. Top with shredded lettuce, diced tomatoes, chopped cilantro, and a dollop of Greek yogurt if desired.
7. Serve immediately.

NUTRIENT CONTENT (PER SERVING):

- Calories: 220
- Total Fat: 10g
- Protein: 6g
- Carbohydrates: 22g
- Sugars: 8g
- Fiber: 9g
- Sodium: 380mg

INGREDIENT TIPS:

- Cauliflower: Low in carbs and calories, high in fiber, and adds a satisfying crunch to the tacos.
- Chickpeas: Provide protein and fiber, making the tacos filling and nutritious.

SPAGHETTI SQUASH PAD THAI

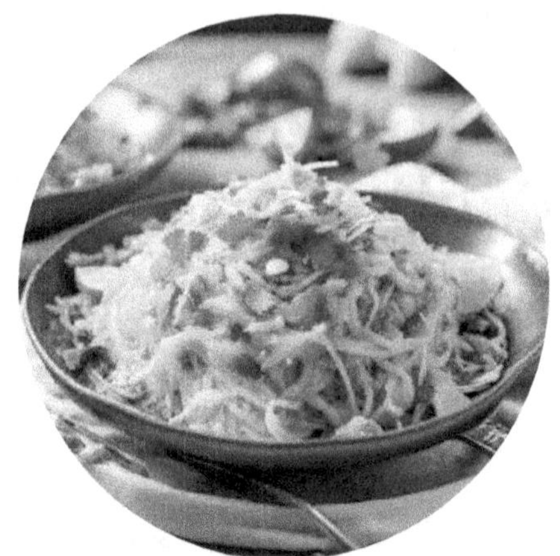

This spaghetti squash pad Thai is a flavorful twist on a classic dish, using spaghetti squash as a low-carb alternative to noodles.

Servings: 4 | Prep Time: 15 minutes | Cook Time: 45 minutes | Carbs per Serving: 25g

INGREDIENTS

- 1 medium spaghetti squash
- 1 tbsp olive oil
- 1 cup tofu, diced
- 2 eggs, beaten
- 1 cup bean sprouts
- 1/2 cup shredded carrots
- 1/4 cup chopped peanuts
- 2 tbsp soy sauce (low sodium)
- 1 tbsp fish sauce (optional)
- 1 tbsp honey or agave syrup
- 1 tbsp lime juice
- 2 cloves garlic, minced
- 1 tsp grated fresh ginger
- 1/4 cup chopped fresh cilantro
- Lime wedges for garnish

DIRECTIONS

1. Preheat oven to 400°F (200°C). Cut spaghetti squash in half lengthwise and remove seeds.
2. Brush squash halves with olive oil and place cut side down on a baking sheet. Roast for 30-40 minutes, until tender.
3. In a large skillet, heat olive oil over medium heat. Add garlic and ginger, sauté for 1 minute.
4. Add diced tofu to the skillet and cook until golden brown.
5. Push tofu to the side and pour beaten eggs into the skillet. Scramble until cooked through.
6. Use a fork to scrape the spaghetti squash strands into the skillet with tofu and eggs.
7. Add bean sprouts, shredded carrots, soy sauce, fish sauce (if using), honey or agave syrup, and lime juice. Stir well to combine and heat through.
8. Garnish with chopped peanuts, fresh cilantro, and lime wedges.

NUTRIENT CONTENT (PER SERVING):

- Calories: 280
- Total Fat: 15g
- Protein: 12g
- Carbohydrates: 25g
- Sugars: 10g
- Fiber: 6g
- Sodium: 420mg

INGREDIENT TIPS:

- Spaghetti Squash: Low in carbs and calories, a great alternative to traditional noodles.
- Tofu: Adds protein and texture to the dish.
- Peanuts: Provides crunch and healthy fats, but use in moderation due to their calorie content.

MEDITERRANEAN CHICKPEA SALAD

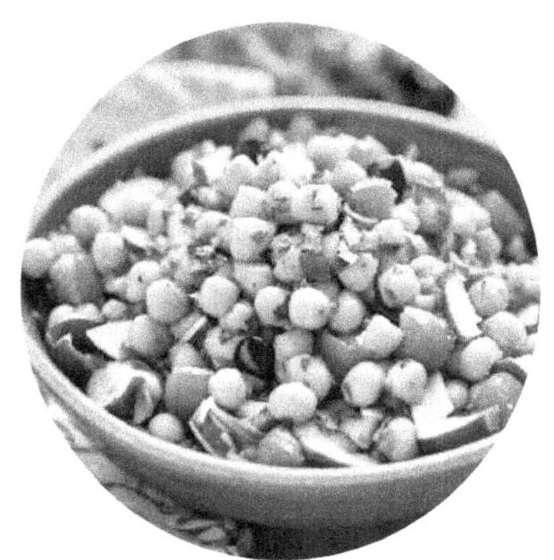

This refreshing Mediterranean chickpea salad is packed with fresh vegetables, herbs, and protein-rich chickpeas, making it a satisfying and diabetes-friendly meal.

Servings: 4 | Prep Time: 15 minutes | Cook Time: 0 minutes | Carbs per Serving: 30g

INGREDIENTS

- 2 cans (15 oz each) chickpeas, drained and rinsed
- 1 cucumber, diced
- 1 cup cherry tomatoes, halved
- 1/2 red onion, thinly sliced
- 1/4 cup chopped fresh parsley
- 1/4 cup chopped fresh mint
- 1/4 cup crumbled feta cheese (optional)
- 1/4 cup Kalamata olives, sliced
- 2 tbsp olive oil
- 1 tbsp red wine vinegar
- 1 tsp dried oregano
- Salt and pepper to taste
- Lemon wedges for garnish

DIRECTIONS

1. In a large bowl, combine chickpeas, cucumber, cherry tomatoes, red onion, parsley, mint, feta cheese (if using), and Kalamata olives.
2. In a small bowl, whisk together olive oil, red wine vinegar, dried oregano, salt, and pepper.
3. Pour dressing over the chickpea mixture and toss to coat evenly.
4. Serve chilled or at room temperature, garnished with lemon wedges.

NUTRIENT CONTENT (PER SERVING):

- Calories: 280
- Total Fat: 10g
- Protein: 10g
- Carbohydrates: 30g
- Sugars: 6g
- Fiber: 8g
- Sodium: 480mg

INGREDIENT TIPS:

- Chickpeas: High in protein and fiber, aiding in blood sugar control.
- Fresh Vegetables and Herbs: Provide essential nutrients and add freshness to the salad.
- **Feta Cheese and Olives**: Add flavor, but use in moderation due to their sodium content.

EGGPLANT PARMESAN

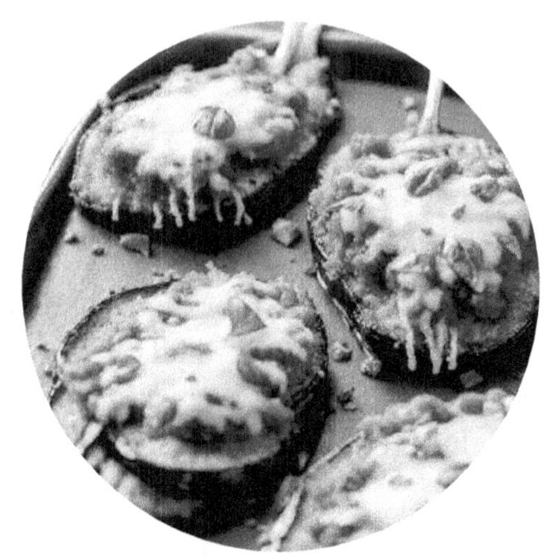

Crispy breaded eggplant slices baked with marinara sauce and melted cheese, a comforting and satisfying meatless dinner option.

Servings: 4 | Prep Time: 20 mins | Cook Time: 25 mins | Carbs per Serving: 20g

INGREDIENTS

- 1 large eggplant, sliced into rounds
- 1 cup breadcrumbs (whole wheat for a healthier option)
- 2 eggs, beaten
- 1 cup marinara sauce
- 1 cup shredded mozzarella cheese
- 1/4 cup grated Parmesan cheese
- Fresh basil leaves for garnish
- Salt and pepper to taste
- Olive oil for frying

DIRECTIONS

1. Preheat oven to 375°F (190°C).
2. Dip eggplant slices in beaten eggs, then coat with breadcrumbs seasoned with salt and pepper.
3. Heat olive oil in a skillet over medium heat.
4. Fry breaded eggplant slices until golden brown on both sides. Drain on paper towels.
5. In a baking dish, spread a layer of marinara sauce.
6. Arrange fried eggplant slices on top of the sauce.
7. Spread more marinara sauce over the eggplant slices.
8. Sprinkle shredded mozzarella cheese and grated Parmesan cheese over the sauce.
9. Repeat layers if desired.
10. Bake in the oven for 20-25 minutes until the cheese is melted and bubbly.
11. Garnish with fresh basil leaves before serving.

NUTRIENT CONTENT (PER SERVING):		INGREDIENT TIPS:
• Calories: 320 • Total Fat: 15g • Protein: 15g • Carbohydrates: 20g	• Sugars: 6g • Fiber: 5g • Sodium: 480mg	Use whole wheat breadcrumbs and low-sodium marinara sauce for a healthier dish. Eggplant provides fiber and nutrients.

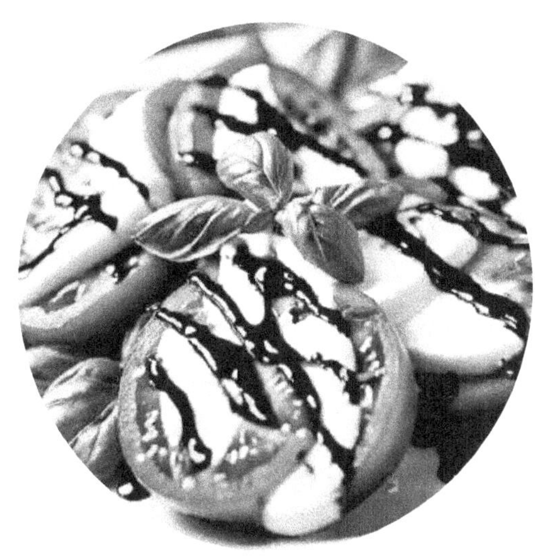

CAPRESE SALAD

A classic and elegant Caprese salad featuring ripe tomatoes, fresh mozzarella, basil, and a drizzle of balsamic glaze, creating a simple yet flavorful dish.

Servings: 4 | Prep Time: 10 mins | Carbs per Serving: 5g

INGREDIENTS

- 2 large tomatoes, sliced
- 1 ball fresh mozzarella cheese, sliced
- Fresh basil leaves
- Balsamic glaze or reduction
- Olive oil
- Salt and pepper to taste

DIRECTIONS

1. Arrange tomato slices and mozzarella slices on a serving platter.
2. Tuck fresh basil leaves between the tomato and cheese slices.
3. Drizzle with balsamic glaze or reduction and olive oil.
4. Season with salt and pepper to taste.
5. Serve immediately as a side dish or appetizer.

NUTRIENT CONTENT (PER SERVING):		INGREDIENT TIPS:
• Calories: 180 • Total Fat: 12g • Protein: 10g • Carbohydrates: 5g	• Sugars: 3g • Fiber: 1g • Sodium: 300mg	Tomatoes offer antioxidants and vitamins. Mozzarella adds creaminess and protein.

CAPRESE STUFFED PORTOBELLO MUSHROOMS

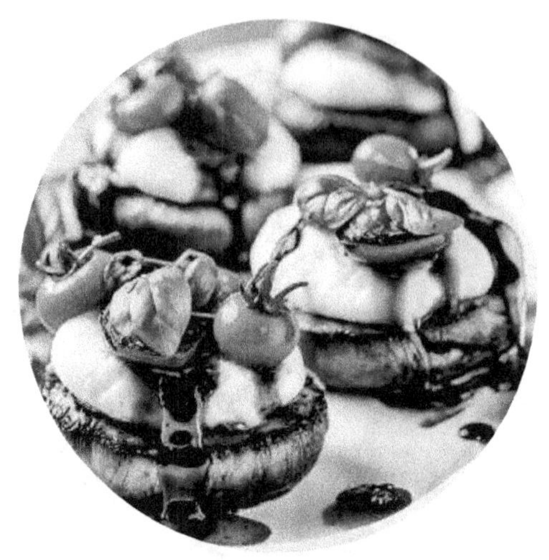

Juicy portobello mushrooms stuffed with a delicious mix of cherry tomatoes, fresh mozzarella, and basil, drizzled with balsamic glaze for a burst of flavor.

Servings: 4 | Prep Time: 15 mins | Cook Time: 15-20 mins | Carbs per Serving: 10g

INGREDIENTS

- 4 large portobello mushrooms, stems removed
- 1 cup cherry tomatoes, halved
- 1 cup fresh mozzarella balls, halved
- 1/4 cup fresh basil leaves, chopped
- 2 tablespoons balsamic glaze
- 2 tablespoons olive oil
- Salt and pepper to taste

DIRECTIONS

1. Preheat oven to 375°F (190°C).
2. Place portobello mushrooms on a baking sheet lined with parchment paper.
3. Drizzle olive oil over the mushrooms and season with salt and pepper.
4. In a bowl, combine cherry tomatoes, mozzarella balls, and chopped basil.
5. Stuff each portobello mushroom with the tomato-mozzarella mixture.
6. Bake in the oven for 15-20 minutes until mushrooms are tender and cheese is melted.
7. Drizzle balsamic glaze over the stuffed mushrooms before serving.

NUTRIENT CONTENT (PER SERVING):		INGREDIENT TIPS:
• Calories: 200 • Total Fat: 12g • Protein: 10g • Carbohydrates: 10g	• Sugars: 6g • Fiber: 3g • Sodium: 180mg	Portobello mushrooms add a meaty texture while tomatoes, mozzarella, and basil create a classic Caprese flavor. Opt for a reduced-sugar balsamic glaze.

VEGETABLE PAELLA

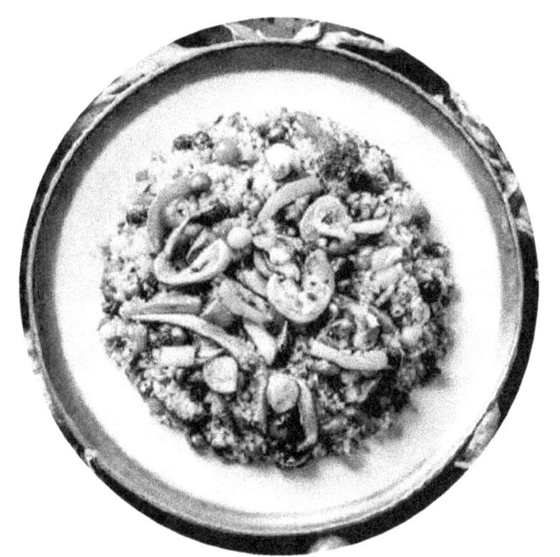

A colorful and flavorful vegetable paella with tender rice, vibrant veggies, and aromatic spices, perfect for a festive meatless meal.

Servings: 4 | Prep Time: 15 mins | Cook Time: 30 mins | Carbs per Serving: 50g

INGREDIENTS

- 1 cup Arborio rice
- 2 cups vegetable broth
- 1 onion, chopped
- 1 bell pepper, diced
- 1 zucchini, sliced
- 1 cup cherry tomatoes, halved
- 1/2 cup frozen peas
- 2 cloves garlic, minced
- 1 teaspoon smoked paprika
- 1/2 teaspoon turmeric
- 1/2 teaspoon saffron threads (optional)
- Salt and pepper to taste
- Olive oil for cooking
- Lemon wedges for serving
- Fresh parsley for garnish

DIRECTIONS

1. Heat olive oil in a large skillet or paella pan over medium heat.
2. Add chopped onion and minced garlic, sauté until softened.
3. Stir in diced bell pepper, sliced zucchini, cherry tomatoes, and frozen peas.
4. Cook vegetables until slightly tender.
5. Add Arborio rice to the pan and toast for a few minutes.
6. Sprinkle smoked paprika, turmeric, saffron threads (if using), salt, and pepper over the rice and vegetables.
7. Pour vegetable broth into the pan and stir well.
8. Bring to a simmer, then reduce heat to low and cover the pan.
9. Cook for 20-25 minutes until rice is tender and liquid is absorbed.
10. Remove from heat and let it sit for 5 minutes before fluffing with a fork.
11. Garnish with fresh parsley and serve with lemon wedges.

NUTRIENT CONTENT (PER SERVING):		INGREDIENT TIPS:
• Calories: 320 • Total Fat: 5g • Protein: 8g • Carbohydrates: 50g	• Sugars: 6g • Fiber: 6g • Sodium: 480mg	Arborio rice creates a creamy texture, and saffron adds authentic flavor. Use low-sodium vegetable broth for a healthier dish.

Chapter Seven

Chicken and Turkey

In the realm of balanced, diabetes-friendly meals, chicken and turkey stand out as lean protein powerhouses that offer versatility and flavor. This chapter, "Chicken and Turkey Recipes for Pre-Diabetic Diet," is crafted with the specific dietary needs of individuals over 50 who are managing pre-diabetes in mind.

As we age, the importance of a nutritious diet becomes even more pronounced, particularly in mitigating the risk of developing type 2 diabetes. Lean poultry like chicken and turkey not only provide essential protein but are also low in saturated fats, making them an ideal choice for maintaining stable blood sugar levels.

Each recipe in this chapter is thoughtfully designed to balance protein with fiber-rich vegetables, whole grains, and spices that enhance flavor without compromising health. From comforting soups and stews to vibrant salads and satisfying main courses, these chicken and turkey dishes offer a delightful array of options to suit various tastes and preferences.

By incorporating these recipes into your pre-diabetic diet, you're not just nourishing your body; you're also embarking on a flavorful journey towards better health and well-being. Let's explore the delicious possibilities that chicken and turkey can bring to your dining table while supporting your efforts to manage pre-diabetes after 50.

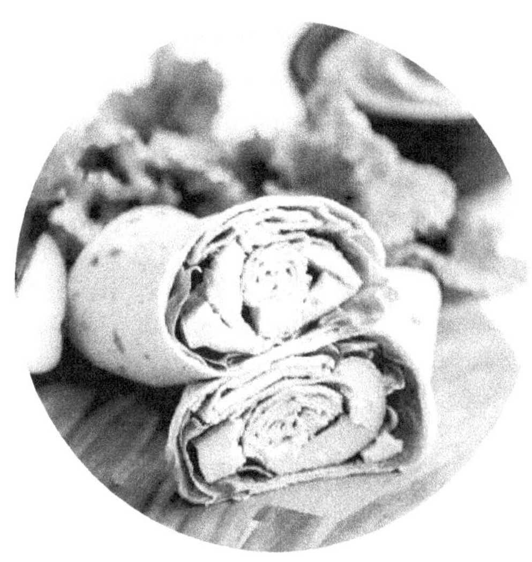

AVOCADO AND TURKEY WRAP

A wholesome and satisfying wrap filled with turkey, avocado, lettuce, and flavorful hummus, perfect for a balanced and delicious lunch.

Servings: 1 | Prep Time: 10 mins | Carbs per Serving: 25g

INGREDIENTS

- 1 whole-grain wrap or tortilla
- 3 ounces sliced turkey breast
- 1/4 avocado, sliced
- 1/4 cup shredded lettuce
- 1/4 cup sliced tomatoes
- 1 tablespoon Greek yogurt or light mayo
- Salt and pepper to taste

DIRECTIONS

1. Lay out the whole-grain wrap on a clean surface.
2. Spread Greek yogurt or light mayo evenly on the wrap.
3. Layer sliced turkey, avocado, lettuce, and tomatoes on top.
4. Season with salt and pepper to taste.
5. Roll up the wrap tightly and slice in half.
6. Secure with toothpicks if needed.
7. Serve immediately or wrap in foil for later.

NUTRIENT CONTENT (PER SERVING):		INGREDIENT TIPS:
• Calories: 320 • Total Fat: 10g • Protein: 20g • Carbohydrates: 25g	• Sugars: 2g • Fiber: 5g • Sodium: 600mg	Whole-grain wraps offer complex carbs and fiber. Avocado adds healthy fats and creaminess.

CHICKEN AND SPINACH STUFFED PORTOBELLO MUSHROOMS

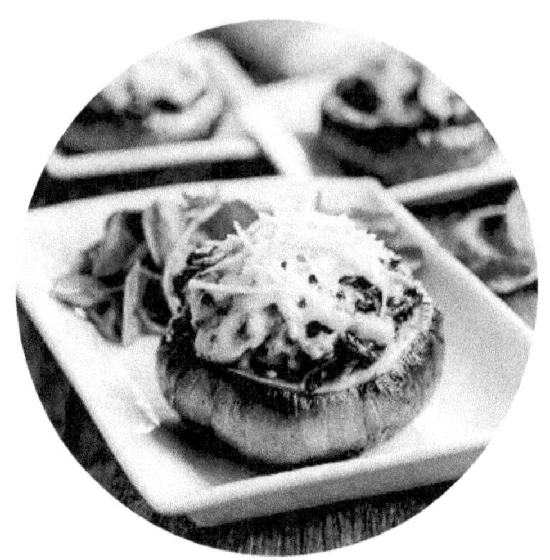

Juicy Portobello mushrooms stuffed with a savory mixture of chicken, spinach, and cheese, a delicious and satisfying dish suitable for lunch or dinner.

Servings: 4 | Prep Time: 15 mins | Cook Time: 20-25 mins | Carbs per Serving: 8g

INGREDIENTS

- 4 large Portobello mushrooms
- 1 lb chicken breast, cooked and shredded
- 2 cups fresh spinach, chopped
- 1/2 cup ricotta cheese
- 1/4 cup grated Parmesan cheese
- 2 cloves garlic, minced
- 1 teaspoon Italian seasoning
- Salt and pepper to taste
- Olive oil for drizzling
- Fresh basil leaves for garnish

DIRECTIONS

1. Preheat the oven to 375°F (190°C).
2. Remove the stems from the Portobello mushrooms and gently scrape out the gills.
3. In a bowl, combine shredded chicken, chopped spinach, ricotta cheese, Parmesan cheese, minced garlic, Italian seasoning, salt, and pepper.
4. Stuff each mushroom cap with the chicken and spinach mixture.
5. Place the stuffed mushrooms on a baking sheet.
6. Drizzle olive oil over the mushrooms.
7. Bake in the preheated oven for 20-25 minutes or until mushrooms are tender and filling is heated through.
8. Garnish with fresh basil leaves before serving.

NUTRIENT CONTENT (PER SERVING):		INGREDIENT TIPS:
• Calories: 280 • Total Fat: 10g • Protein: 35g • Carbohydrates: 8g	• Sugars: 2g • Fiber: 2g • Sodium: 320mg	Opt for lean chicken breast and low-fat ricotta for a healthier option. Feel free to add chopped sun-dried tomatoes for extra flavor.

TURKEY AND LENTIL STUFFED BELL PEPPERS

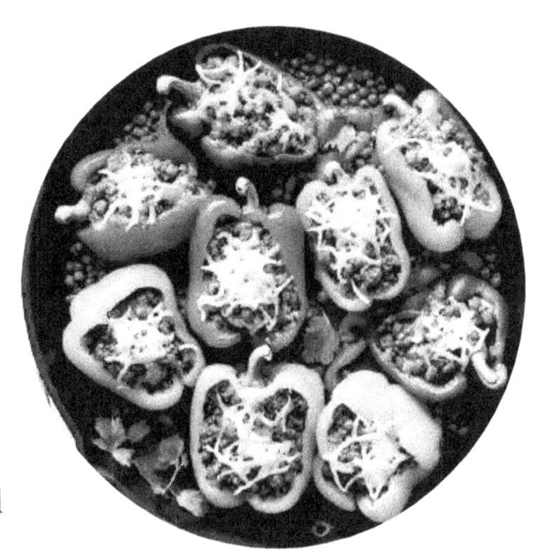

Colorful bell peppers filled with a hearty mixture of turkey, lentils, and spices, topped with melted cheese for a nutritious and flavorful meal option.

Servings: 4 | Prep Time: 20 mins | Cook Time: 40 mins | Carbs per Serving: 20g

INGREDIENTS

- 4 large bell peppers (any color)
- 1 lb ground turkey
- 1 cup cooked lentils
- 1 onion, finely chopped
- 2 cloves garlic, minced
- 1 teaspoon cumin powder
- 1 teaspoon paprika
- Salt and pepper to taste
- 1 cup tomato sauce
- Shredded mozzarella cheese for topping
- Fresh parsley for garnish

DIRECTIONS

1. Preheat the oven to 375°F (190°C).
2. Cut the tops off the bell peppers and remove the seeds and membranes.
3. In a skillet, cook ground turkey until browned. Add chopped onions and minced garlic, cook until onions are translucent.
4. Stir in cooked lentils, cumin powder, paprika, salt, and pepper. Cook for a few more minutes.
5. Fill each bell pepper with the turkey and lentil mixture.
6. Place the stuffed peppers in a baking dish.
7. Pour tomato sauce over the stuffed peppers.
8. Cover the dish with foil and bake for 30-35 minutes.
9. Remove foil, sprinkle shredded mozzarella cheese on top of each pepper, and bake for an additional 5 minutes or until cheese is melted and bubbly.
10. Garnish with fresh parsley before serving.

NUTRIENT CONTENT (PER SERVING):		INGREDIENT TIPS:
• Calories: 320 • Total Fat: 10g • Protein: 30g • Carbohydrates: 20g	• Sugars: 8g • Fiber: 6g • Sodium: 480mg	Use cooked lentils for added fiber and protein. Customize the filling with your favorite herbs and spices.

LEMON GARLIC ROAST CHICKEN THIGHS

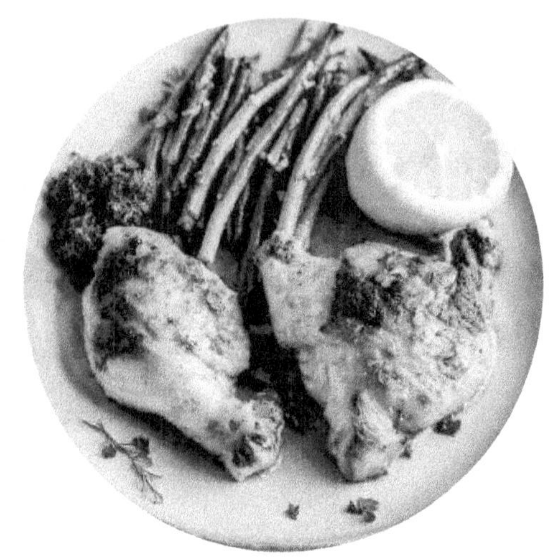

Tender and succulent roast chicken thighs infused with zesty lemon and aromatic garlic, a simple yet elegant dish suitable for any dinner occasion.

Servings: 4 | Prep Time: 10 mins | Cook Time: 30-35 mins | Carbs per Serving: 0g

INGREDIENTS

- 4 chicken thighs, bone-in and skin-on
- Zest and juice of 1 lemon
- 3 tablespoons olive oil
- 4 cloves garlic, minced
- 1 tablespoon chopped fresh rosemary
- Salt and pepper to taste

DIRECTIONS

1. Preheat the oven to 400°F (200°C).
2. In a bowl, combine lemon zest, lemon juice, olive oil, minced garlic, chopped fresh rosemary, salt, and pepper.
3. Place chicken thighs in a baking dish.
4. Pour the lemon garlic mixture over the chicken thighs, ensuring they are coated evenly.
5. Roast in the preheated oven for 30-35 minutes or until chicken is golden and cooked through.
6. Remove from the oven and let rest for a few minutes before serving.

NUTRIENT CONTENT (PER SERVING):		INGREDIENT TIPS:
• Calories: 320 • Total Fat: 20g • Protein: 30g • Carbohydrates: 0g	• Sugars: 0g • Fiber: 0g • Sodium: 140mg	Use bone-in, skin-on chicken thighs for juicier and more flavorful results. Adjust cooking time if using boneless thighs.

CHICKEN AND SPINACH ALFREDO PASTA

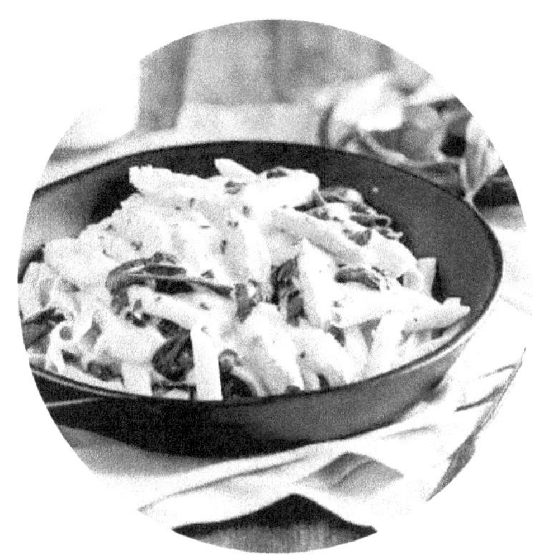

Creamy and indulgent pasta dish featuring tender chicken strips, fresh spinach, and a rich Alfredo sauce, perfect for a comforting family meal.

Servings: 4 | Prep Time: 15 mins | Cook Time: 20 mins | Carbs per Serving: 40g

INGREDIENTS

- 1 lb boneless, skinless chicken breast, cut into strips
- 8 oz fettuccine pasta
- 2 cups fresh spinach leaves
- 1 cup heavy cream
- 1/2 cup grated Parmesan cheese
- 2 tablespoons butter
- 2 cloves garlic, minced
- Salt and pepper to taste
- Fresh parsley for garnish

DIRECTIONS

1. Cook fettuccine pasta according to package instructions until al dente. Drain and set aside.
2. In a skillet, melt butter over medium heat. Add minced garlic and cook until fragrant.
3. Add chicken strips to the skillet and cook until browned and cooked through.
4. Stir in heavy cream and grated Parmesan cheese. Cook until the sauce thickens slightly.
5. Add fresh spinach leaves to the skillet and cook until wilted.
6. Season the sauce with salt and pepper to taste.
7. Add the cooked fettuccine to the skillet and toss to coat with the creamy sauce.
8. Garnish with fresh parsley before serving.

NUTRIENT CONTENT (PER SERVING):		INGREDIENT TIPS:
• Calories: 450 • Total Fat: 22g • Protein: 35g • Carbohydrates: 40g	• Sugars: 3g • Fiber: 3g • Sodium: 280mg	Use whole wheat pasta for added fiber. You can also add sun-dried tomatoes or mushrooms for extra flavor.

TURKEY AND QUINOA STUFFED BELL PEPPERS

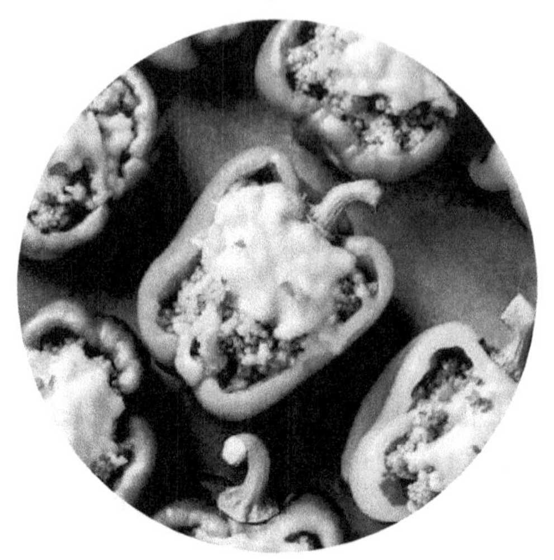

Flavorful bell peppers stuffed with a hearty mixture of turkey, quinoa, and spices, topped with melted cheddar cheese for a satisfying and nutritious meal option.

Servings: 4 | Prep Time: 20 mins | Cook Time: 40 mins | Carbs per Serving: 30g

INGREDIENTS

- 4 large bell peppers (any color)
- 1 lb ground turkey
- 1 cup cooked quinoa
- 1 onion, finely chopped
- 2 cloves garlic, minced
- 1 teaspoon chili powder
- 1 teaspoon ground cumin
- Salt and pepper to taste
- 1 cup tomato sauce
- Shredded cheddar cheese for topping
- Fresh cilantro for garnish

DIRECTIONS

1. Preheat the oven to 375°F (190°C).
2. Cut the tops off the bell peppers and remove the seeds and membranes.
3. In a skillet, cook ground turkey until browned. Add chopped onions and minced garlic, cook until onions are translucent.
4. Stir in cooked quinoa, chili powder, ground cumin, salt, and pepper. Cook for a few more minutes.
5. Fill each bell pepper with the turkey and quinoa mixture.
6. Place the stuffed peppers in a baking dish.
7. Pour tomato sauce over the stuffed peppers.
8. Cover the dish with foil and bake for 30-35 minutes.
9. Remove foil, sprinkle shredded cheddar cheese on top of each pepper, and bake for an additional 5 minutes or until cheese is melted and bubbly.
10. Garnish with fresh cilantro before serving.

NUTRIENT CONTENT (PER SERVING):	INGREDIENT TIPS:
• Calories: 380 • Total Fat: 15g • Protein: 30g • Carbohydrates: 30g • Sugars: 8g • Fiber: 6g • Sodium: 450mg	Feel free to add diced tomatoes or black beans to the filling for added texture and flavor

LEMON HERB ROASTED CHICKEN BREAST

This Lemon Herb Roasted Chicken Breast is a flavorful and protein-packed dish that's perfect for balancing glucose levels and supporting a pre-diabetic diet. The combination of fresh herbs and zesty lemon creates a delicious meal that's both nutritious and satisfying.

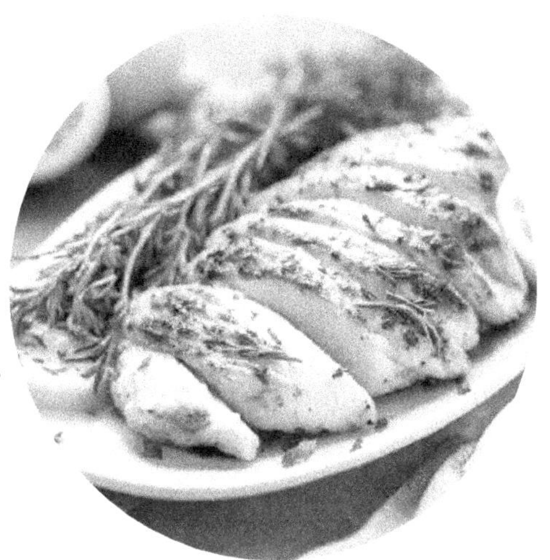

Servings: 4 | Prep Time: 10 minutes | Cook Time: 25 minutes | Carbs per Serving: 1g

INGREDIENTS

- 4 boneless, skinless chicken breasts
- 2 tbsp olive oil
- 2 tbsp fresh lemon juice
- 2 cloves garlic, minced
- 1 tsp dried thyme
- 1 tsp dried rosemary
- 1 tsp dried oregano
- Salt and pepper to taste
- Lemon slices for garnish

DIRECTIONS

1. Preheat oven to 400°F (200°C).
2. In a small bowl, whisk together olive oil, lemon juice, minced garlic, dried thyme, rosemary, oregano, salt, and pepper.
3. Place chicken breasts in a baking dish and pour the marinade over them, ensuring they are evenly coated.
4. Bake for 20-25 minutes or until chicken is cooked through and internal temperature reaches 165°F (75°C).
5. Garnish with lemon slices and fresh herbs before serving.

NUTRIENT CONTENT (PER SERVING):

- Calories: 220
- Total Fat: 10g
- Protein: 30g
- Carbohydrates: 1g
- Sugars: 0g
- Fiber: 0g
- Sodium: 350mg

INGREDIENT TIPS:

- Chicken Breast: Low in saturated fat and high in protein, making it an excellent choice for blood sugar management.
- Herbs: Fresh herbs like thyme, rosemary, and oregano add flavor without extra calories or carbohydrates.

TURKEY AND VEGETABLE STIR-FRY

This Turkey and Vegetable Stir-Fry is a colorful and nutrient-packed dish that's quick to prepare and perfect for balancing blood sugar levels. Loaded with lean protein and fiber-rich vegetables, it's a delicious way to support a pre-diabetic diet.

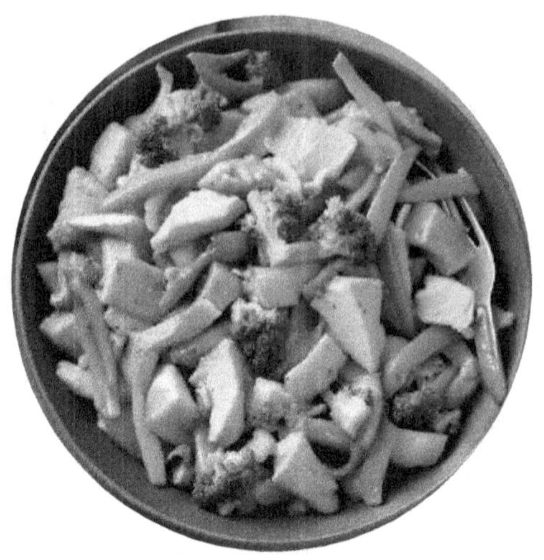

Servings: 4 | Prep Time: 10 minutes | Cook Time: 15 minutes | Carbs per Serving: 8g

INGREDIENTS

- 1 lb lean ground turkey
- 2 cups mixed vegetables (bell peppers, broccoli, carrots)
- 1 tbsp olive oil
- 2 cloves garlic, minced
- 1 tbsp soy sauce (low sodium)
- 1 tsp sesame oil
- 1 tsp ginger, grated
- Salt and pepper to taste
- Green onions for garnish

DIRECTIONS

1. Heat olive oil in a large skillet or wok over medium-high heat.
2. Add minced garlic and grated ginger, sauté for 1 minute until fragrant.
3. Add ground turkey to the skillet and cook until browned.
4. Add mixed vegetables and stir-fry until tender-crisp.
5. Stir in soy sauce, sesame oil, salt, and pepper. Cook for an additional 2-3 minutes.
6. Garnish with chopped green onions before serving

NUTRIENT CONTENT (PER SERVING):

- Calories: 280
- Total Fat: 15g
- Protein: 25g
- Carbohydrates: 8g
- Sugars: 3g
- Fiber: 3g
- Sodium: 380mg

INGREDIENT TIPS:

- Ground Turkey: Lean protein source, low in saturated fat and beneficial for blood sugar control.
- Mixed Vegetables: Fiber-rich and low in calories, providing essential nutrients and aiding in digestion.

GRILLED LEMON HERB TURKEY CUTLETS

These Grilled Lemon Herb Turkey Cutlets are bursting with flavor and make for a light yet satisfying meal. The combination of citrusy lemon and aromatic herbs adds zest to lean turkey cutlets, creating a dish that's perfect for managing blood sugar levels.

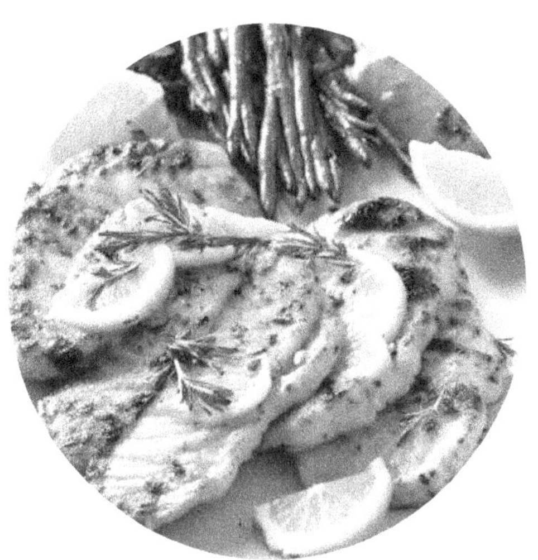

Servings: 4 | Prep Time: 5 minutes | Cook Time: 10 minutes | Carbs per Serving: 1g

INGREDIENTS

- 1 lb turkey cutlets
- 2 tbsp olive oil
- 2 tbsp fresh lemon juice
- 1 tsp dried thyme
- 1 tsp dried rosemary
- Salt and pepper to taste
- Lemon wedges for garnish
- Fresh parsley for garnish

DIRECTIONS

1. Preheat grill or grill pan over medium-high heat.
2. In a small bowl, combine olive oil, lemon juice, dried thyme, dried rosemary, salt, and pepper.
3. Brush both sides of turkey cutlets with the marinade.
4. Grill turkey cutlets for 4-5 minutes per side or until cooked through and grill marks appear.
5. Garnish with lemon wedges and fresh parsley before serving.

NUTRIENT CONTENT (PER SERVING):

- Calories: 180
- Total Fat: 8g
- Protein: 25g
- Carbohydrates: 1g
- Sugars: 0g
- Fiber: 0g
- Sodium: 320mg

INGREDIENT TIPS:

- Turkey Cutlets: Lean protein option that's low in saturated fat and suitable for blood sugar management.
- Lemon: Adds brightness and vitamin C, enhancing the flavor without adding extra calories or carbs.

CHICKEN AND QUINOA SALAD WITH LEMON VINAIGRETTE

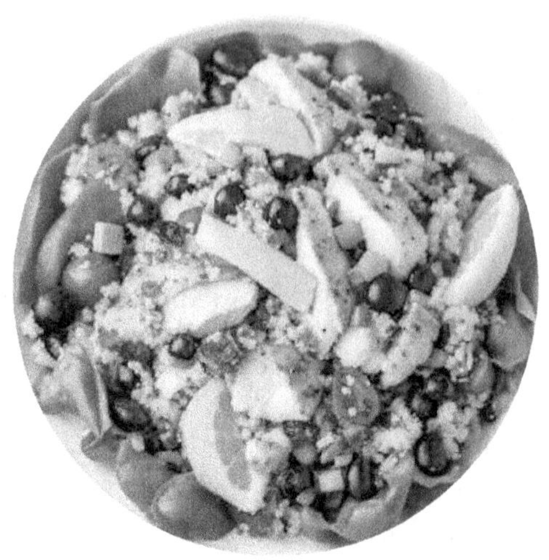

This Chicken and Quinoa Salad with Lemon Vinaigrette is a refreshing and nutrient-rich meal that's perfect for balancing glucose levels and supporting a pre-diabetic diet. Packed with protein, fiber, and healthy fats, it's a delicious and satisfying option.

Servings: 4 | Prep Time: 15 minutes | Cook Time: 15 minutes | Carbs per Serving: 25g

INGREDIENTS

- 1 lb boneless, skinless chicken breasts
- 1 cup quinoa, cooked
- 2 cups mixed greens (spinach, arugula, kale)
- 1 cup cherry tomatoes, halved
- 1 cucumber, diced
- 1/4 cup red onion, thinly sliced
- 1/4 cup feta cheese, crumbled (optional)
- 1/4 cup chopped fresh parsley
- 1/4 cup olive oil
- 2 tbsp fresh lemon juice
- 1 tsp Dijon mustard
- 1 clove garlic, minced
- Salt and pepper to taste

DIRECTIONS

1. Season chicken breasts with salt and pepper.
2. Grill or pan-sear chicken until cooked through, about 6-7 minutes per side. Let it rest before slicing.
3. In a large bowl, combine cooked quinoa, mixed greens, cherry tomatoes, cucumber, red onion, and crumbled feta cheese (if using).
4. In a small bowl, whisk together olive oil, lemon juice, Dijon mustard, minced garlic, salt, and pepper to make the vinaigrette.
5. Pour the vinaigrette over the salad ingredients and toss to coat evenly.
6. Slice grilled chicken and place on top of the salad.
7. Garnish with chopped fresh parsley before serving.

NUTRIENT CONTENT (PER SERVING):

- Calories: 350
- Total Fat: 18g
- Protein: 28g
- Carbohydrates: 25g
- Sugars: 3g
- Fiber: 4g
- Sodium: 320mg

INGREDIENT TIPS:

- Chicken Breasts: Lean protein source that's low in saturated fat, perfect for blood sugar control.
- Quinoa: Complex carb with a low glycemic index, providing sustained energy and fiber.

TURKEY AND VEGETABLE SKEWERS

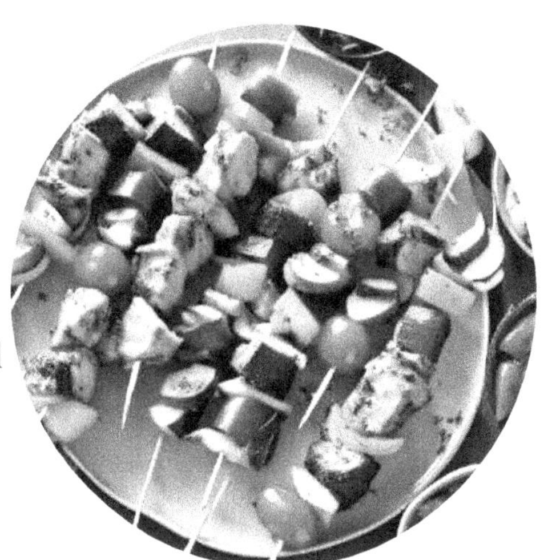

These Turkey and Vegetable Skewers are a colorful and flavorful way to enjoy a balanced meal. Packed with lean protein and fiber-rich veggies, they're perfect for managing blood sugar levels and supporting a pre-diabetic diet.

Servings: 4 | Prep Time: 20 minutes | Cook Time: 10 minutes | Carbs per Serving: 8g

INGREDIENTS

- 1 lb turkey breast, cut into cubes
- 1 zucchini, sliced
- 1 bell pepper, cut into chunks
- 1 red onion, cut into wedges
- 8 cherry tomatoes
- 2 tbsp olive oil
- 2 tbsp balsamic vinegar
- 1 tsp dried Italian seasoning
- Salt and pepper to taste
- Wooden skewers, soaked in water

DIRECTIONS

1. Preheat grill or grill pan over medium-high heat.
2. Thread turkey cubes, zucchini slices, bell pepper chunks, red onion wedges, and cherry tomatoes onto the soaked wooden skewers.
3. In a small bowl, whisk together olive oil, balsamic vinegar, dried Italian seasoning, salt, and pepper to make the marinade.
4. Brush the marinade over the skewers, coating them evenly.
5. Grill skewers for 8-10 minutes, turning occasionally, until turkey is cooked through and veggies are tender.
6. Serve hot.

NUTRIENT CONTENT (PER SERVING):

- Calories: 280
- Total Fat: 10g
- Protein: 30g
- Carbohydrates: 8g
- Sugars: 4g
- Fiber: 2g
- Sodium: 320mg

INGREDIENT TIPS:

- Turkey Breast: Lean protein choice that's low in saturated fat and supports stable blood sugar.
- Vegetables: Zucchini, bell peppers, red onion, and cherry tomatoes add color, nutrients, and fiber to the skewers.

LEMON GARLIC CHICKEN AND BROCCOLI STIR-FRY

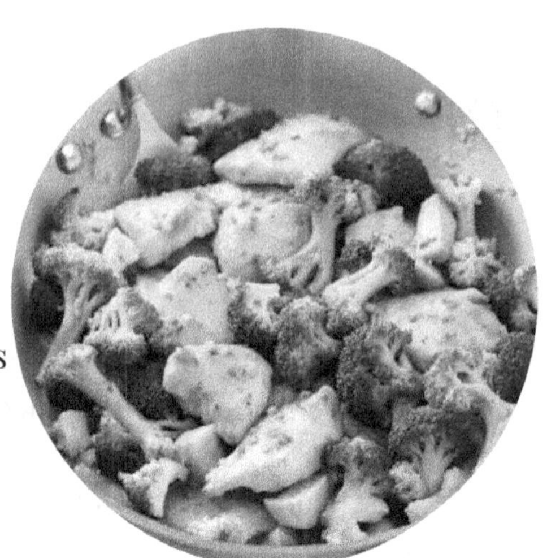

This Lemon Garlic Chicken and Broccoli Stir-Fry is a quick and delicious meal that's perfect for busy weeknights. Loaded with lean protein and fiber-rich broccoli, it's a great choice for balancing glucose levels and supporting a pre-diabetic diet.

Servings: 4 | Prep Time: 10 minutes | Cook Time: 15 minutes | Carbs per Serving: 10g

INGREDIENTS

- 1 lb boneless, skinless chicken thighs, cut into strips
- 2 cups broccoli florets
- 2 tbsp olive oil
- 3 cloves garlic, minced
- 2 tbsp fresh lemon juice
- 1 tsp lemon zest
- 1 tbsp soy sauce (low sodium)
- 1 tsp honey or agave syrup
- Salt and pepper to taste
- Red pepper flakes (optional)
- Sesame seeds for garnish

DIRECTIONS

1. Heat olive oil in a large skillet or wok over medium-high heat.
2. Add minced garlic and red pepper flakes (if using), sauté for 1 minute until fragrant.
3. Add chicken strips to the skillet and cook until browned and cooked through.
4. Add broccoli florets to the skillet and stir-fry for 3-4 minutes until tender-crisp.
5. In a small bowl, whisk together fresh lemon juice, lemon zest, soy sauce, honey or agave syrup, salt, and pepper to make the sauce.
6. Pour the sauce over the chicken and broccoli in the skillet. Stir well to coat everything evenly.
7. Cook for an additional 2-3 minutes until the sauce thickens slightly and coats the chicken and broccoli.
8. Remove from heat and garnish with sesame seeds before serving.

NUTRIENT CONTENT (PER SERVING):		INGREDIENT TIPS:
• Calories: 280 • Total Fat: 14g • Protein: 25g • Carbohydrates: 10g	• Sugars: 4g • Fiber: 3g • Sodium: 350mg	• Chicken Thighs: Provide juicy, flavorful protein with slightly higher fat content than chicken breasts. • Broccoli: Fiber-rich vegetable that adds texture, nutrients, and helps regulate blood sugar levels.

MEDITERRANEAN TURKEY MEATBALLS WITH ZUCCHINI NOODLES

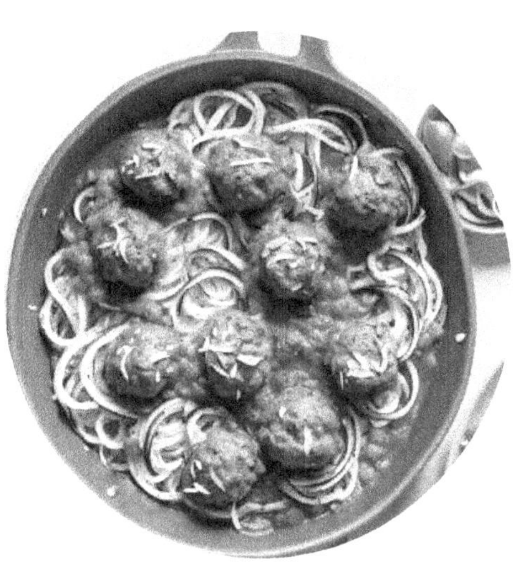

These Mediterranean Turkey Meatballs with Zucchini Noodles are a delicious and low-carb alternative to traditional pasta dishes. Packed with lean protein and veggies, they're perfect for maintaining stable blood sugar levels.

Servings: 4 | Prep Time: 15 minutes | Cook Time: 20 minutes | Carbs per Serving: 10g

INGREDIENTS

- 1 lb lean ground turkey
- 1/2 cup almond flour
- 1/4 cup grated Parmesan cheese
- 1 egg
- 2 cloves garlic, minced
- 1 tbsp dried oregano
- 1 tsp dried basil
- Salt and pepper to taste
- 2 tbsp olive oil
- 2 cups zucchini noodles (zoodles)
- 1 cup marinara sauce (sugar-free)
- Fresh basil leaves for garnish

DIRECTIONS

1. In a large bowl, combine ground turkey, almond flour, Parmesan cheese, egg, minced garlic, dried oregano, dried basil, salt, and pepper. Mix until well combined.
2. Form the mixture into meatballs, about 1 inch in diameter.
3. Heat olive oil in a skillet over medium heat. Add meatballs and cook until browned on all sides and cooked through.
4. Remove meatballs from the skillet and set aside.
5. In the same skillet, add zucchini noodles and sauté for 2-3 minutes until tender.
6. Return meatballs to the skillet, add marinara sauce, and gently toss to coat everything.
7. Cook for an additional 2-3 minutes until heated through.
8. Serve hot, garnished with fresh basil leaves.

NUTRIENT CONTENT (PER SERVING):		INGREDIENT TIPS:
• Calories: 320 • Total Fat: 18g • Protein: 25g • Carbohydrates: 10g	• Sugars: 4g • Fiber: 3g • Sodium: 420mg	• Ground Turkey: Lean protein base for the meatballs, providing satiety and blood sugar stability. • Almond Flour: Low-carb alternative to breadcrumbs, adding texture and healthy fats.

Chapter Eight

BEEF, PORK, AND LAMB

This chapter in the "Pre-Diabetic Diet Cookbook and Meal Plan After 50" is dedicated to helping you discover delicious and health-conscious ways to enjoy these protein-rich meats while keeping your blood sugar levels in check.

Navigating a pre-diabetic diet can feel daunting, but with the right ingredients and culinary techniques, you can create meals that are both satisfying and supportive of your health goals. Lean cuts of beef, pork, and lamb offer essential nutrients like iron, zinc, and protein without excessive saturated fats, making them valuable additions to a balanced diet aimed at preventing or managing diabetes.

Each recipe in this chapter is thoughtfully crafted to balance protein with fiber-rich vegetables, whole grains, and flavorful spices. From hearty stews and comforting roasts to creative stir-fries and nutritious salads, you'll find a variety of options to suit your taste preferences and dietary needs.

By exploring these recipes, you'll not only discover new ways to enjoy beef, pork, and lamb but also gain insights into how to create meals that promote stable blood sugar levels and overall well-being. Let's embark on a culinary journey that nourishes your body and supports your journey toward a healthier lifestyle after 50.

LAMB CURRY WITH CAULIFLOWER RICE

A fragrant and comforting lamb curry served with cauliflower rice, a low-carb and flavorful alternative to traditional rice.

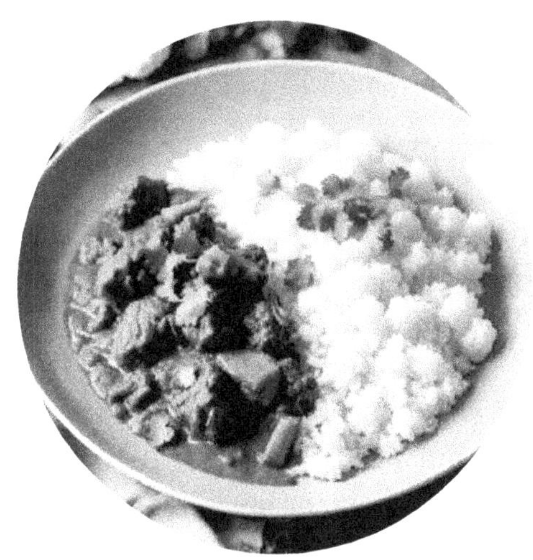

Servings: 4 | Prep Time: 20 mins | Cook Time: 1 hour 15 mins | Carbs per Serving: 15g

INGREDIENTS

- 1 lb lamb stew meat, cubed
- 1 onion, chopped
- 2 cloves garlic, minced
- 1 tablespoon grated ginger
- 1 tablespoon curry powder
- 1 can (14 oz) diced tomatoes
- 1 can (14 oz) coconut milk
- 1 head cauliflower, grated or processed into rice-like texture
- 2 tablespoons olive oil
- Fresh cilantro for garnish
- Salt and pepper to taste

DIRECTIONS

1. In a large pot or Dutch oven, heat olive oil over medium heat.
2. Add chopped onion and sauté until translucent.
3. Add minced garlic, grated ginger, and curry powder. Cook for a minute until fragrant.
4. Add cubed lamb to the pot and brown on all sides.
5. Pour in diced tomatoes and coconut milk. Stir well to combine.
6. Bring the curry to a simmer, then reduce heat to low and cover. Let it simmer for about 1 hour or until lamb is tender.
7. While the curry simmers, prepare the cauliflower rice by grating or processing cauliflower into rice-like texture.
8. Heat a separate pan with a little olive oil. Add cauliflower rice and sauté until tender.
9. Season cauliflower rice with salt and pepper.
10. Serve the lamb curry hot over cauliflower rice, garnished with fresh cilantro.

NUTRIENT CONTENT (PER SERVING):		INGREDIENT TIPS:
• Calories: 400 • Total Fat: 25g • Protein: 25g • Carbohydrates: 15g	• Sugars: 5g • Fiber: 5g • Sodium: 450mg	Choose lean lamb stew meat and adjust curry powder according to spice preference.

BEEF AND VEGETABLE STIR-FRY WITH QUINOA

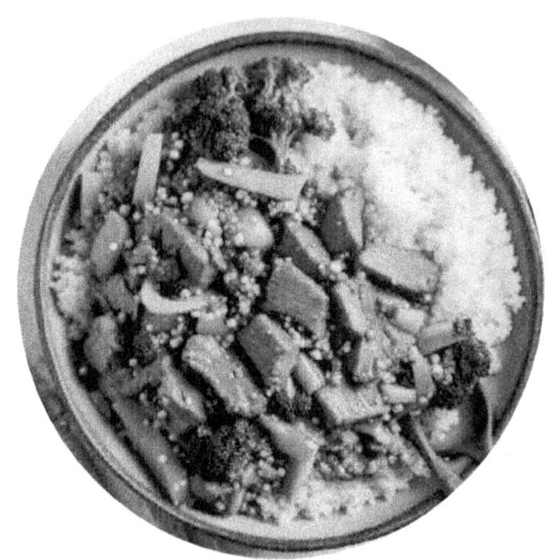

A flavorful beef and vegetable stir-fry served over nutritious quinoa, a satisfying and balanced meal for busy weeknights.

Servings: 4 | Prep Time: 15 mins | Cook Time: 15 mins | Carbs per Serving: 30g

INGREDIENTS

- 1 lb beef sirloin, thinly sliced
- 1 cup broccoli florets
- 1 cup sliced carrots
- 1 red bell pepper, sliced
- 1 yellow bell pepper, sliced
- 1 onion, sliced
- 2 cloves garlic, minced
- 1 teaspoon grated ginger
- 2 tablespoons soy sauce (low-sodium)
- 1 tablespoon hoisin sauce
- 1 tablespoon cornstarch
- 2 tablespoons olive oil
- Cooked quinoa for serving

DIRECTIONS

1. In a small bowl, mix soy sauce, hoisin sauce, cornstarch, and grated ginger. Set aside.
2. Heat olive oil in a wok or large skillet over high heat.
3. Add minced garlic to the skillet and stir-fry for a few seconds until fragrant.
4. Add sliced beef and stir-fry until browned. Remove beef from the skillet and set aside.
5. In the same skillet, add more oil if needed and stir-fry broccoli, carrots, bell peppers, and onion until crisp-tender.
6. Return the cooked beef to the skillet.
7. Pour the soy sauce mixture over the beef and vegetables. Stir well to coat everything evenly and cook for a minute until the sauce thickens.
8. Serve hot over cooked quinoa.

NUTRIENT CONTENT (PER SERVING):		INGREDIENT TIPS:
• Calories: 400	• Sugars: 5g	Opt for lean beef cuts like sirloin for a healthier stir-fry. Quinoa adds protein and fiber to the dish.
• Total Fat: 15g	• Fiber: 5g	
• Protein: 30g	• Sodium: 600mg	
• Carbohydrates: 30g		

PORK CHOPS WITH BALSAMIC GLAZE

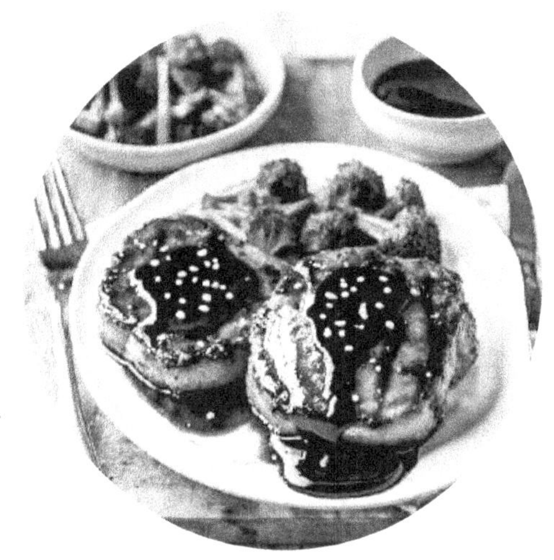

Juicy and tender pork chops glazed with a sweet and tangy balsamic sauce, a delightful dish that's easy to make yet impressive enough for special occasions.

Servings: 4 | Prep Time: 10 mins | Cook Time: 15 mins | Carbs per Serving: 15g

INGREDIENTS

- 4 pork loin chops
- Salt and pepper to taste
- 2 tablespoons olive oil
- 1/4 cup balsamic vinegar
- 2 tablespoons honey or maple syrup
- 2 cloves garlic, minced
- Fresh thyme for garnish

DIRECTIONS

1. Season pork chops with salt and pepper on both sides.
2. In a skillet, heat olive oil over medium-high heat.
3. Add pork chops to the skillet and cook for about 4-5 minutes per side or until fully cooked and browned.
4. Remove pork chops from the skillet and set aside.
5. In the same skillet, add minced garlic and sauté until fragrant.
6. Pour in balsamic vinegar and honey or maple syrup. Stir well to combine.
7. Simmer the glaze for a few minutes until it thickens slightly.
8. Return the pork chops to the skillet, coating them with the balsamic glaze.
9. Cook for another minute to heat through.
10. Garnish with fresh thyme before serving.

NUTRIENT CONTENT (PER SERVING):		INGREDIENT TIPS:
• Calories: 350 • Total Fat: 15g • Protein: 25g • Carbohydrates: 15g	• Sugars: 10g • Fiber: 1g • Sodium: 350mg	Choose lean pork loin chops for this recipe. Adjust sweetness by varying the amount of honey or maple syrup used.

GRILLED LAMB CHOPS WITH MINT CHIMICHURRI

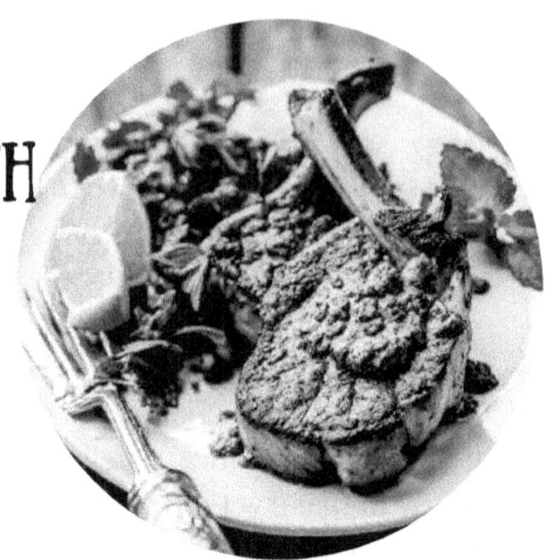

Juicy grilled lamb chops infused with a refreshing mint chimichurri sauce, perfect for a flavorful and elegant dinner.

Servings: 4 | Prep Time: 10 mins | Cook Time: 8 mins | Carbs per Serving: 0g

INGREDIENTS

- 8 lamb loin chops
- Salt and pepper to taste
- 2 tablespoons olive oil
- Fresh mint leaves for garnish

Mint Chimichurri:
- 1 cup fresh mint leaves, chopped
- 1/4 cup fresh parsley leaves, chopped
- 2 cloves garlic, minced
- 1/4 cup olive oil
- 2 tablespoons red wine vinegar
- Salt and pepper to taste

DIRECTIONS

1. Preheat the grill to medium-high heat.
2. Season lamb chops with salt, pepper, and olive oil.
3. Grill lamb chops for about 3-4 minutes per side for medium-rare doneness.
4. Remove lamb chops from the grill and let them rest for a few minutes.
5. Meanwhile, prepare the mint chimichurri by combining chopped mint leaves, parsley, minced garlic, olive oil, red wine vinegar, salt, and pepper in a bowl. Mix well.
6. Serve grilled lamb chops hot, topped with mint chimichurri sauce and garnished with fresh mint leaves.

NUTRIENT CONTENT (PER SERVING):
- Calories: 350
- Total Fat: 15g
- Protein: 25g
- Carbohydrates: 15g
- Sugars: 10g
- Fiber: 1g
- Sodium: 350mg

INGREDIENT TIPS:

Use fresh herbs for the chimichurri sauce for the best flavor. Lamb loin chops are ideal for grilling due to their tenderness.

PORK TENDERLOIN WITH MAPLE GLAZE

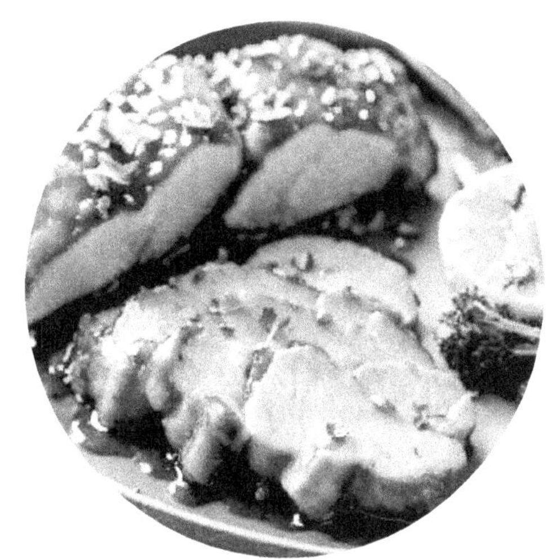

Tender and juicy pork tenderloin coated in a sweet and savory maple glaze, a simple yet impressive dish that's perfect for any occasion.

Servings: 4 | Prep Time: 10 mins | Cook Time: 25 mins | Carbs per Serving: 10g

INGREDIENTS

- 1 lb pork tenderloin
- Salt and pepper to taste
- 2 tablespoons olive oil
- 1/4 cup maple syrup
- 2 tablespoons Dijon mustard
- 1 tablespoon apple cider vinegar
- 2 cloves garlic, minced
- Fresh rosemary for garnish

DIRECTIONS

1. Preheat the oven to 400°F (200°C).
2. Season pork tenderloin with salt and pepper.
3. Heat olive oil in an oven-safe skillet over medium-high heat.
4. Sear the pork tenderloin on all sides until browned.
5. In a small bowl, mix maple syrup, Dijon mustard, apple cider vinegar, minced garlic, salt, and pepper.
6. Pour the maple glaze mixture over the seared pork tenderloin in the skillet.
7. Transfer the skillet to the preheated oven and roast for about 15-20 minutes or until pork reaches an internal temperature of 145°F (63°C).
8. Remove the pork tenderloin from the oven and let it rest for a few minutes before slicing.
9. Garnish with fresh rosemary before serving.

NUTRIENT CONTENT (PER SERVING):		INGREDIENT TIPS:
• Calories: 350 • Total Fat: 15g • Protein: 25g • Carbohydrates: 15g	• Sugars: 10g • Fiber: 1g • Sodium: 350mg	Choose pure maple syrup for the glaze for the best flavor. Pork tenderloin is a lean and tender cut that cooks quickly.

BEEF STIR-FRY WITH BROCCOLI AND BROWN RICE

A flavorful and balanced meal that's perfect for managing blood sugar levels. The combination of lean beef, fiber-rich broccoli, and complex carbs from brown rice creates a satisfying dish that supports a pre-diabetic diet.

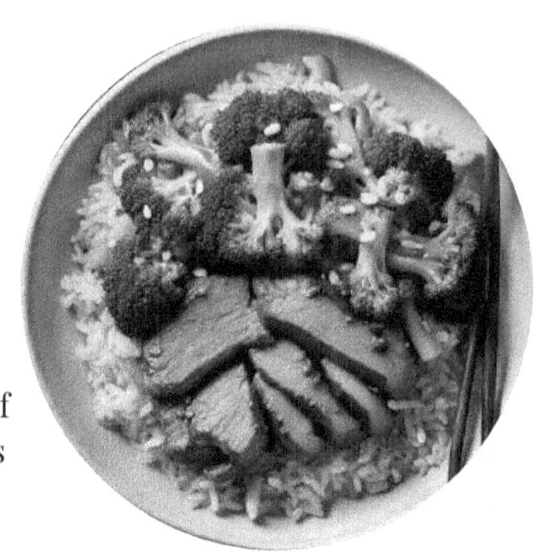

Servings: 4 | Prep Time: 15 minutes | Cook Time: 15 minutes | Carbs per Serving: 30g

INGREDIENTS

- 1 lb lean beef sirloin, thinly sliced
- 2 cups broccoli florets
- 1 cup cooked brown rice
- 2 tbsp low-sodium soy sauce
- 1 tbsp olive oil
- 2 cloves garlic, minced
- 1 tsp grated fresh ginger
- Salt and pepper to taste
- Red pepper flakes (optional)
- Green onions for garnish

DIRECTIONS

1. In a bowl, marinate beef slices with soy sauce, minced garlic, grated ginger, salt, pepper, and optional red pepper flakes.
2. Heat olive oil in a skillet or wok over medium-high heat.
3. Add marinated beef to the skillet and stir-fry until browned and cooked through.
4. Add broccoli florets to the skillet and continue stir-frying until tender-crisp.
5. Serve the beef and broccoli over cooked brown rice.
6. Garnish with chopped green onions before serving.

NUTRIENT CONTENT (PER SERVING):

- Calories: 320
- Total Fat: 10g
- Protein: 30g
- Carbohydrates: 30g
- Sugars: 3g
- Fiber: 5g
- Sodium: 480mg

INGREDIENT TIPS:

- Beef Sirloin: Lean protein source that's low in saturated fat and rich in iron.
- Broccoli: Fiber-rich vegetable that aids in digestion and blood sugar control.
- Brown Rice: Complex carbohydrate with a lower glycemic index compared to white rice.

PORK TENDERLOIN WITH ROASTED VEGETABLES

This Pork Tenderloin with Roasted Vegetables is a hearty and nutritious dish that's perfect for managing blood sugar levels. The combination of tender pork, colorful veggies, and flavorful herbs creates a satisfying meal that supports a pre-diabetic diet.

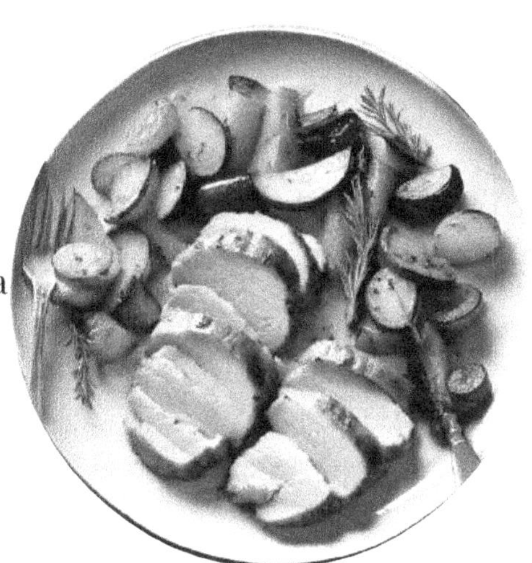

Servings: 4 | Prep Time: 10 minutes | Cook Time: 30 minutes | Carbs per Serving: 15g

INGREDIENTS

- 1 lb pork tenderloin
- 2 cups mixed vegetables (bell peppers, zucchini, carrots)
- 1 tbsp olive oil
- 1 tsp dried thyme
- 1 tsp dried rosemary
- 1 tsp paprika
- Salt and pepper to taste
- Lemon wedges for garnish

DIRECTIONS

1. Preheat oven to 400°F (200°C).
2. Season pork tenderloin with dried thyme, dried rosemary, paprika, salt, and pepper.
3. Place pork tenderloin in a roasting pan and surround it with mixed vegetables.
4. Drizzle olive oil over the pork and vegetables.
5. Roast in the oven for 25-30 minutes or until pork is cooked through and veggies are tender.
6. Let the pork rest before slicing.
7. Serve pork slices with roasted vegetables and garnish with lemon wedges.

NUTRIENT CONTENT (PER SERVING):

- Calories: 280
- Total Fat: 10g
- Protein: 30g
- Carbohydrates: 15g
- Sugars: 5g
- Fiber: 5g
- Sodium: 420mg

INGREDIENT TIPS:

- Pork Tenderloin: Lean cut of pork that's low in fat and high in protein.
- Mixed Vegetables: Colorful assortment of veggies adds vitamins, minerals, and fiber to the dish.
- Herbs and Spices: Dried thyme, rosemary, and paprika add flavor without extra calories or sodium.

LAMB AND CHICKPEA CURRY

This Lamb and Chickpea Curry is a fragrant and comforting dish that's packed with protein and fiber. The combination of tender lamb, creamy chickpeas, and aromatic spices creates a flavorful meal that supports stable blood sugar levels.

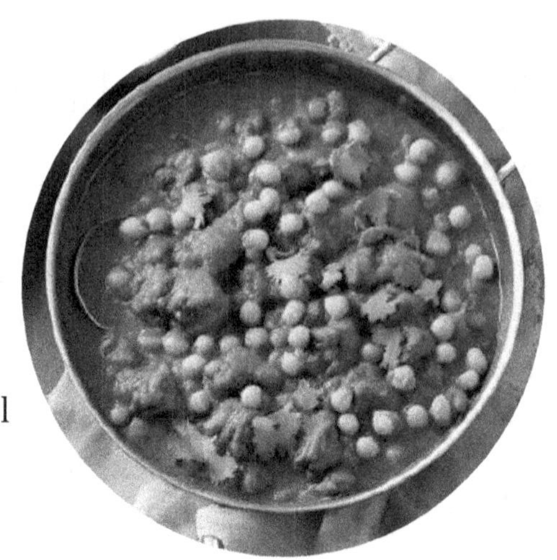

Servings: 4 | Prep Time: 15 minutes | Cook Time: 2 hours | Carbs per Serving: 20g

INGREDIENTS

- 1 lb lamb stew meat, cubed
- 1 can (15 oz) chickpeas, drained and rinsed
- 1 onion, chopped
- 2 cloves garlic, minced
- 1 tbsp olive oil
- 1 can (14 oz) diced tomatoes
- 1 cup low-sodium chicken broth
- 2 tsp curry powder
- 1 tsp ground cumin
- 1 tsp ground coriander
- Salt and pepper to taste
- Fresh cilantro for garnish

DIRECTIONS

1. In a large pot or Dutch oven, heat olive oil over medium heat.
2. Add chopped onion and minced garlic, sauté until softened.
3. Add cubed lamb stew meat to the pot and brown on all sides.
4. Stir in curry powder, ground cumin, ground coriander, salt, and pepper.
5. Add diced tomatoes, chicken broth, and drained chickpeas to the pot.
6. Bring to a boil, then reduce heat and simmer for 1.5-2 hours until lamb is tender.
7. Serve the lamb and chickpea curry hot, garnished with fresh cilantro.

NUTRIENT CONTENT (PER SERVING):	INGREDIENT TIPS:
• Calories: 380 • Total Fat: 15g • Protein: 35g • Carbohydrates: 20g • Sugars: 5g • Fiber: 7g • Sodium: 480mg	• Lamb Stew Meat: Provides protein, iron, and flavor to the curry. • Chickpeas: High in fiber and protein, aiding in blood sugar control and satiety. • Spices: Curry powder, cumin, and coriander add depth of flavor without excessive sodium.

BEEF AND VEGETABLE SKEWERS WITH QUINOA

These Beef and Vegetable Skewers with Quinoa are a delightful and nutritious option for a balanced meal. Lean beef combined with colorful veggies and quinoa provides protein, fiber, and complex carbs that are beneficial for blood sugar management.

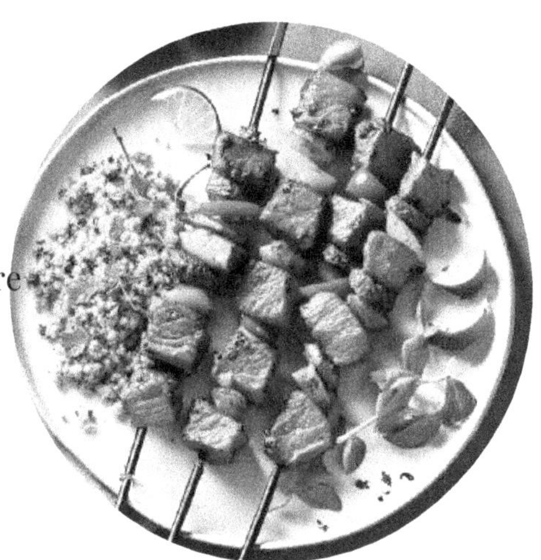

Servings: 4 | Prep Time: 20 minutes | Cook Time: 10 minutes Carbs per Serving: 25g

INGREDIENTS

- 1 lb beef sirloin, cut into cubes
- 2 bell peppers (red, yellow), cut into chunks
- 1 red onion, cut into wedges
- 1 zucchini, sliced
- 1 cup cooked quinoa
- 2 tbsp olive oil
- 2 tbsp balsamic vinegar
- 1 tsp dried Italian seasoning
- Salt and pepper to taste
- Wooden skewers, soaked in water

DIRECTIONS

1. Preheat grill or grill pan over medium-high heat.
2. Thread beef cubes, bell pepper chunks, onion wedges, and zucchini slices onto soaked wooden skewers.
3. In a small bowl, whisk together olive oil, balsamic vinegar, Italian seasoning, salt, and pepper to make the marinade.
4. Brush the marinade over the skewers, coating them evenly.
5. Grill skewers for 8-10 minutes, turning occasionally, until beef is cooked to desired doneness and veggies are tender.
6. Serve skewers over cooked quinoa.

NUTRIENT CONTENT (PER SERVING):

- Calories: 350
- Total Fat: 15g
- Protein: 30g
- Carbohydrates: 25g
- Sugars: 4g
- Fiber: 4g
- Sodium: 320mg

INGREDIENT TIPS:

- Beef Sirloin: Lean protein choice with essential nutrients like iron and B vitamins.
- Bell Peppers and Zucchini: Colorful veggies that contribute vitamins, minerals, and fiber to the dish.
- Quinoa: Provides complex carbs and additional protein, aiding in blood sugar stability.

PORK AND BEAN CHILI

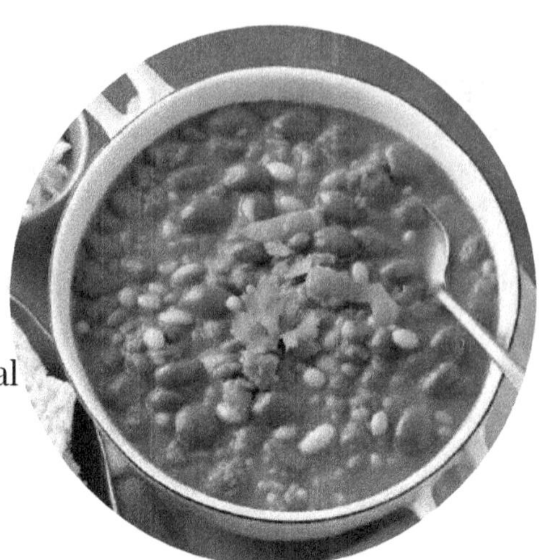

This Pork and Bean Chili is a hearty and flavorful dish that's perfect for cooler days. Loaded with lean pork, beans, and spices, it's a comforting meal that supports blood sugar management while providing essential nutrients.

Servings: 6 | Prep Time: 15 minutes | Cook Time: 40 minutes | Carbs per Serving: 25g

INGREDIENTS

- 1 lb lean ground pork
- 1 can (15 oz) kidney beans, drained and rinsed
- 1 can (15 oz) black beans, drained and rinsed
- 1 can (14 oz) diced tomatoes
- 1 onion, chopped
- 2 cloves garlic, minced
- 1 tbsp olive oil
- 2 tbsp chili powder
- 1 tsp ground cumin
- Salt and pepper to taste
- Fresh cilantro for garnish
- Greek yogurt (optional topping)

DIRECTIONS

1. In a large pot or Dutch oven, heat olive oil over medium heat.
2. Add chopped onion and minced garlic, sauté until softened.
3. Add ground pork to the pot and cook until browned.
4. Stir in chili powder, ground cumin, salt, and pepper.
5. Add diced tomatoes, kidney beans, and black beans to the pot. Stir well.
6. Bring to a simmer, then reduce heat and cook for 30-40 minutes, stirring occasionally.
7. Serve the chili hot, garnished with fresh cilantro and a dollop of Greek yogurt if desired.

NUTRIENT CONTENT (PER SERVING):

- Calories: 320
- Total Fat: 10g
- Protein: 25g
- Carbohydrates: 25g
- Sugars: 5g
- Fiber: 8g
- Sodium: 480mg

INGREDIENT TIPS:

- Lean Ground Pork: Provides protein and flavor without excessive fat.
- Beans: Kidney beans and black beans are rich in fiber and protein, aiding in blood sugar control and satiety.
- Spices: Chili powder and cumin add warmth and depth of flavor to the chili.

Chapter Nine

FISH AND SEAFOOD

This collection of fish and seafood recipes is crafted to support individuals over 50 in managing pre-diabetes and promoting overall health through delicious and nutritious meals.

Fish and seafood are nutritional powerhouses, rich in omega-3 fatty acids, lean protein, and essential vitamins and minerals. Incorporating these ingredients into your diet can help regulate blood sugar levels, reduce inflammation, and support heart health—all vital aspects of a pre-diabetic diet.

In this chapter, you'll discover a variety of recipes that celebrate the flavors of the sea while prioritizing ingredients that promote stable glucose levels. From succulent grilled fish to flavorful seafood stews, each dish is designed with your well-being in mind.

Whether you're a seafood enthusiast or looking to explore new culinary horizons, these recipes offer a delightful way to nourish your body and enjoy meals that are both beneficial and enjoyable. Let's embark on a journey of vibrant flavors and healthful choices that elevate your dining experience while supporting your pre-diabetic diet goals.

CREAMY GARLIC SHRIMP PASTA

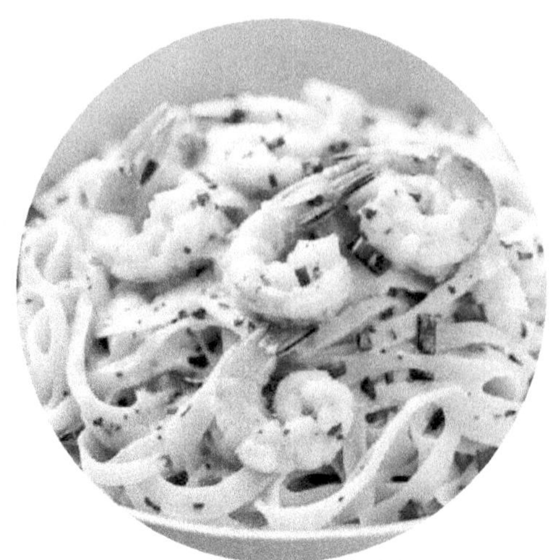

Rich and creamy garlic shrimp pasta tossed with fettuccine, a comforting and decadent dish that's sure to please pasta lovers.

Servings: 4 | Prep Time: 10 mins | Cook Time: 15 mins | Carbs per Serving: 45g

INGREDIENTS

- 1 lb shrimp, peeled and deveined
- Salt and pepper to taste
- 8 oz fettuccine pasta
- 2 tablespoons olive oil
- 4 cloves garlic, minced
- 1 cup heavy cream
- 1/2 cup grated Parmesan cheese
- 1 tablespoon fresh parsley, chopped
- Lemon zest for garnish

DIRECTIONS

1. Cook fettuccine pasta according to package instructions. Drain and set aside.
2. Season shrimp with salt and pepper.
3. In a skillet, heat olive oil over medium heat.
4. Add minced garlic to the skillet and sauté until fragrant.
5. Add seasoned shrimp to the skillet and cook for about 2-3 minutes per side or until pink and cooked through.
6. Pour heavy cream into the skillet and bring to a simmer.
7. Stir in grated Parmesan cheese until melted and creamy.
8. Add cooked fettuccine pasta to the creamy sauce and toss to coat evenly.
9. Stir in chopped parsley.
10. Serve hot with a sprinkle of lemon zest on top.

NUTRIENT CONTENT (PER SERVING):	INGREDIENT TIPS:
- Calories: 550 - Total Fat: 32g - Protein: 35g - Carbohydrates: 45g - Sugars: 3g - Fiber: 2g - Sodium: 350mg	Creamy garlic shrimp pasta is indulgent yet satisfying. Use fresh parsley and lemon zest for a burst of flavor.

LEMON HERB BAKED COD

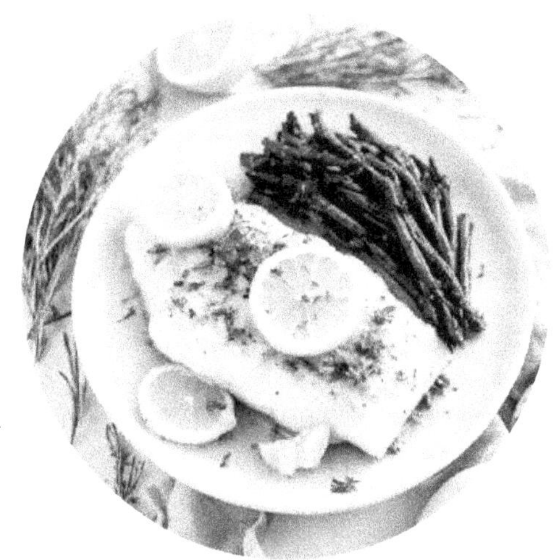

Tender baked cod infused with zesty lemon and aromatic herbs, a simple yet flavorful seafood dish that's perfect for a healthy dinner.

Servings: 4 | Prep Time: 10 mins | Cook Time: 15-20 mins | Carbs per Serving: 2g

INGREDIENTS

- 4 cod fillets
- Salt and pepper to taste
- 2 tablespoons olive oil
- Juice of 1 lemon
- 2 tablespoons fresh parsley, chopped
- 1 teaspoon dried thyme
- 1 teaspoon dried oregano
- 1 teaspoon garlic powder
- Lemon wedges for serving

DIRECTIONS

1. Preheat the oven to 400°F (200°C) and grease a baking dish with olive oil.
2. Place the cod fillets in the baking dish and season with salt and pepper.
3. In a small bowl, mix together olive oil, lemon juice, chopped parsley, dried thyme, dried oregano, and garlic powder.
4. Drizzle the herb mixture over the cod fillets, ensuring they are evenly coated.
5. Bake in the preheated oven for about 15-20 minutes or until the fish flakes easily with a fork.
6. Remove from the oven and garnish with additional fresh parsley and lemon wedges.
7. Serve hot with a side of steamed vegetables or quinoa.

NUTRIENT CONTENT (PER SERVING):		INGREDIENT TIPS:
• Calories: 200 • Total Fat: 9g • Protein: 27g • Carbohydrates: 2g	• Sugars: 0g • Fiber: 1g • Sodium: 120mg	The combination of lemon and herbs adds a burst of freshness to the mild-flavored cod. Adjust the seasoning according to your preference.

SPICY GRILLED SHRIMP TACOS

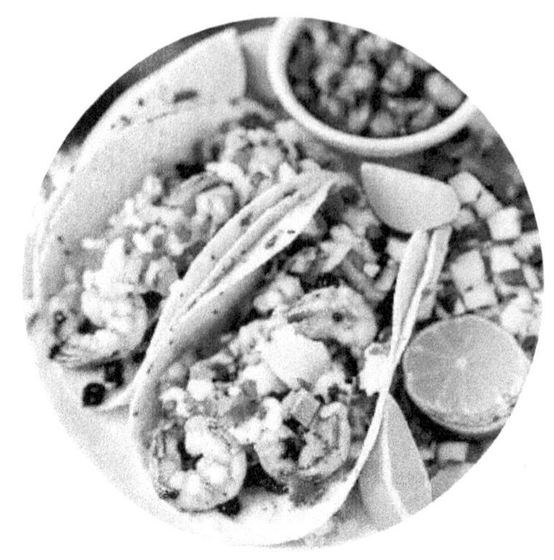

Spicy grilled shrimp tacos with a medley of fresh toppings, a flavorful and satisfying meal that's perfect for taco night or a quick weeknight dinner.

Servings: 4 | Prep Time: 15 mins | Cook Time: 6-8 mins | Carbs per Serving: 20g

INGREDIENTS

- 1 lb large shrimp, peeled and deveined
- Salt and pepper to taste
- 1 tablespoon olive oil
- 1 teaspoon chili powder
- 1/2 teaspoon paprika
- 1/2 teaspoon cumin
- 1/4 teaspoon garlic powder
- 1/4 teaspoon onion powder
- 1/4 teaspoon cayenne pepper (optional for extra spice)
- 8 small corn tortillas
- Sliced avocado, shredded cabbage, diced tomatoes, and lime wedges for serving

DIRECTIONS

1. Preheat the grill or grill pan over medium-high heat.
2. In a bowl, toss shrimp with olive oil, salt, pepper, chili powder, paprika, cumin, garlic powder, onion powder, and cayenne pepper (if using).
3. Thread seasoned shrimp onto skewers.
4. Grill shrimp skewers for about 2-3 minutes per side or until shrimp are pink and slightly charred.
5. Warm corn tortillas on the grill for about 30 seconds per side.
6. Assemble tacos by placing grilled shrimp, sliced avocado, shredded cabbage, and diced tomatoes on each tortilla.
7. Squeeze fresh lime juice over the tacos.
8. Serve hot with your favorite salsa or hot sauce on the side.

NUTRIENT CONTENT (PER SERVING):	INGREDIENT TIPS:
• Calories: 300 • Total Fat: 8g • Protein: 25g • Carbohydrates: 20g • Sugars: 1g • Fiber: 4g • Sodium: 350mg	Customize your tacos with your favorite toppings like salsa, sour cream, or cheese. Adjust the spice level of the shrimp marinade to your liking.

COCONUT LIME SHRIMP CURRY

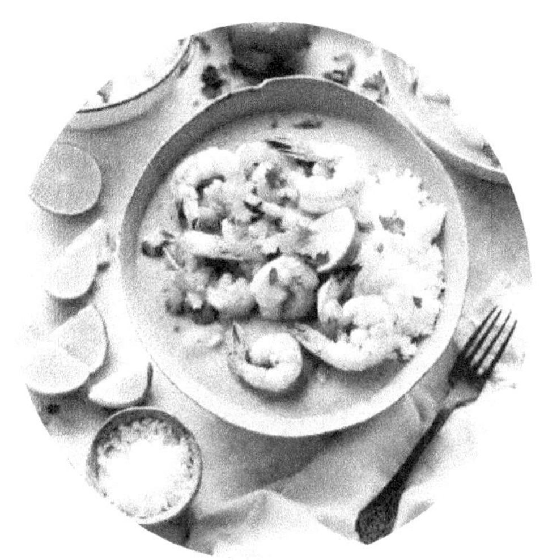

Aromatic coconut lime shrimp curry with a hint of spice, perfect for a comforting and satisfying meal served over rice or cauliflower rice.

Servings: 4 | Prep Time: 15 mins | Cook Time: 15 mins | Carbs per Serving: 10g

INGREDIENTS

- 1 lb large shrimp, peeled and deveined
- Salt and pepper to taste
- 2 tablespoons coconut oil
- 1 onion, chopped
- 3 cloves garlic, minced
- 1 tablespoon ginger, grated
- 2 tablespoons curry powder
- 1 can (14 oz) coconut milk
- Juice and zest of 1 lime
- 1 tablespoon fish sauce
- Fresh cilantro for garnish
- Cooked rice or cauliflower rice for serving

DIRECTIONS

1. Season shrimp with salt and pepper.
2. In a large skillet, heat coconut oil over medium heat.
3. Add chopped onion, minced garlic, and grated ginger to the skillet. Sauté until onions are translucent.
4. Stir in curry powder and cook for another minute until fragrant.
5. Add shrimp to the skillet and cook for about 2-3 minutes per side or until shrimp are pink and cooked through.
6. Pour in coconut milk, lime juice, lime zest, and fish sauce. Stir to combine and let it simmer for 5-7 minutes.
7. Adjust seasoning with salt and pepper if needed.
8. Serve hot over cooked rice or cauliflower rice.
9. Garnish with fresh cilantro before serving.

NUTRIENT CONTENT (PER SERVING):		INGREDIENT TIPS:
• Calories: 350 • Total Fat: 23g • Protein: 25g • Carbohydrates: 10g	• Sugars: 2g • Fiber: 2g • Sodium: 450mg	Coconut milk adds a creamy texture while lime juice adds a zesty kick to this flavorful shrimp curry. Adjust the spice level by adding more or less curry powder.

MEDITERRANEAN GRILLED SWORDFISH

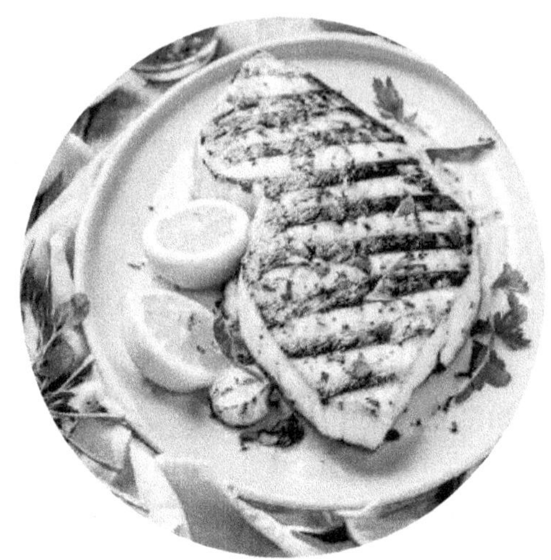

Grilled swordfish infused with Mediterranean flavors of lemon, garlic, and herbs, a delicious and healthy seafood dish that's perfect for summer grilling.

Servings: 4 | Prep Time: 10 mins | Marinating Time: 30 mins | Cook Time: 8-10 mins | Carbs per Serving: 1g

INGREDIENTS

- 4 swordfish steaks
- Salt and pepper to taste
- 2 tablespoons olive oil
- Juice of 1 lemon
- 2 cloves garlic, minced
- 1 teaspoon dried oregano
- 1 teaspoon dried basil
- 1/2 teaspoon paprika
- Lemon wedges and fresh parsley for garnish

DIRECTIONS

1. Season swordfish steaks with salt and pepper.
2. In a bowl, whisk together olive oil, lemon juice, minced garlic, dried oregano, dried basil, and paprika to create the marinade.
3. Place swordfish steaks in a shallow dish and pour the marinade over them. Ensure the steaks are evenly coated.
4. Let the swordfish marinate for at least 30 minutes in the refrigerator.
5. Preheat the grill to medium-high heat.
6. Grill swordfish steaks for about 4-5 minutes per side or until fish is cooked through and has grill marks.
7. Remove from the grill and garnish with lemon wedges and fresh parsley.
8. Serve hot with a side of grilled vegetables or a quinoa salad

NUTRIENT CONTENT (PER SERVING):		INGREDIENT TIPS:
• Calories: 300 • Total Fat: 15g • Protein: 35g • Carbohydrates: 1g	• Sugars: 0g • Fiber: 0g • Sodium: 180mg	Swordfish has a meaty texture and pairs well with Mediterranean flavors like lemon, garlic, and herbs. Adjust grilling time based on the thickness of the steaks.

GRILLED SALMON WITH LEMON HERB BUTTER

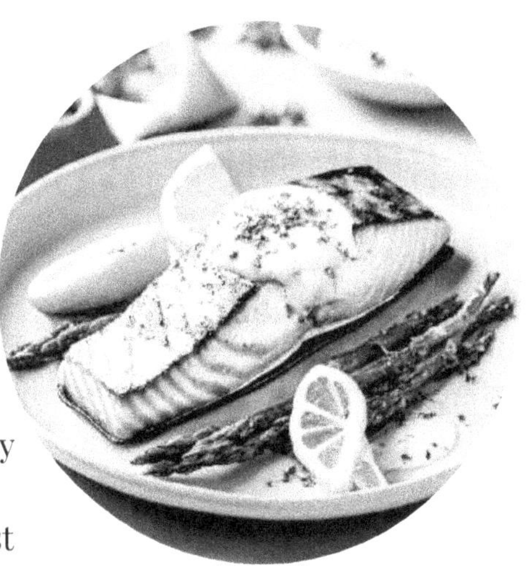

This Grilled Salmon with Lemon Herb Butter is a flavorful and nutritious dish that's perfect for managing blood sugar levels. Rich in omega-3 fatty acids and protein, salmon provides essential nutrients while the lemon herb butter adds a burst of flavor.

Servings: 4 | Prep Time: 10 minutes | Cook Time: 10 minutes | Carbs per Serving: 0g

INGREDIENTS

- 4 salmon fillets
- 2 tbsp unsalted butter, softened
- 1 tbsp fresh lemon juice
- 1 tsp lemon zest
- 1 tbsp chopped fresh dill
- Salt and pepper to taste
- Lemon slices for garnish

DIRECTIONS

1. Preheat grill to medium-high heat.
2. In a bowl, combine softened butter, lemon juice, lemon zest, chopped dill, salt, and pepper to make the lemon herb butter.
3. Season salmon fillets with salt and pepper.
4. Grill salmon for 4-5 minutes per side or until cooked to desired doneness.
5. Remove salmon from grill and top each fillet with a dollop of lemon herb butter.
6. Garnish with lemon slices before serving.

NUTRIENT CONTENT (PER SERVING):

- Calories: 250
- Total Fat: 14g
- Protein: 28g
- Carbohydrates: 0g
- Sugars: 0g
- Fiber: 0g
- Sodium: 120mg

INGREDIENT TIPS:

- Salmon: Rich in omega-3 fatty acids and protein, salmon supports heart health and stable blood sugar levels.
- Lemon Herb Butter: Adds flavor without added sugars or carbs, enhancing the taste of the grilled salmon.

SHRIMP AND AVOCADO SALAD

This Shrimp and Avocado Salad is a refreshing and light meal that's perfect for a balanced diet. With protein-packed shrimp, healthy fats from avocado, and a zesty dressing, it's a flavorful option for managing blood sugar levels.

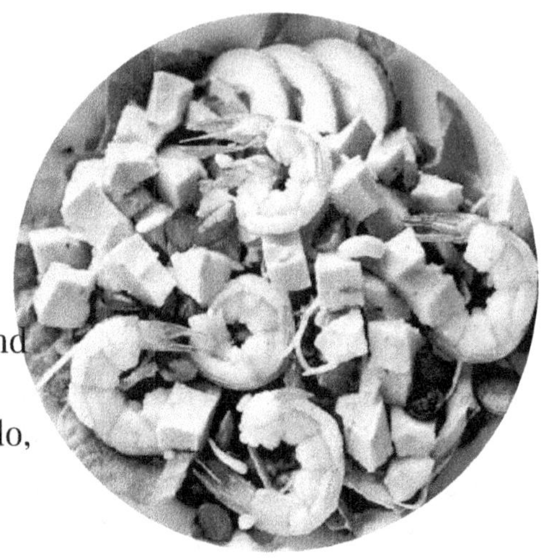

Servings: 4 | Prep Time: 15 minutes | Cook Time: 5 minutes | Carbs per Serving: 10g

INGREDIENTS

- 1 lb shrimp, peeled and deveined
- 2 avocados, diced
- 1 cup cherry tomatoes, halved
- 1/4 cup chopped red onion
- 2 tbsp olive oil
- 1 tbsp fresh lime juice
- 1 tsp honey or agave syrup
- Salt and pepper to taste
- Fresh cilantro for garnish

DIRECTIONS

1. In a bowl, whisk together olive oil, lime juice, honey or agave syrup, salt, and pepper to make the dressing.
2. Season shrimp with salt and pepper.
3. Heat a skillet over medium-high heat and cook shrimp for 2-3 minutes per side until pink and cooked through.
4. In a large salad bowl, combine diced avocado, cherry tomatoes, chopped red onion, and cooked shrimp.
5. Drizzle the dressing over the salad and toss gently to coat.
6. Garnish with fresh cilantro before serving.

NUTRIENT CONTENT (PER SERVING):

- Calories: 280
- Total Fat: 18g
- Protein: 25g
- Carbohydrates: 10g
- Sugars: 4g
- Fiber: 5g
- Sodium: 320mg

INGREDIENT TIPS:

- Shrimp: Low in calories and high in protein, shrimp is a lean seafood option for blood sugar management.
- Avocado: Provides healthy fats, fiber, and potassium, contributing to satiety and heart health.

BAKED COD WITH ROASTED VEGETABLES

This Baked Cod with Roasted Vegetables is a simple yet satisfying dish that's packed with nutrients. Cod is a lean protein source, while roasted veggies add fiber and vitamins, making it an ideal choice for a pre-diabetic diet.

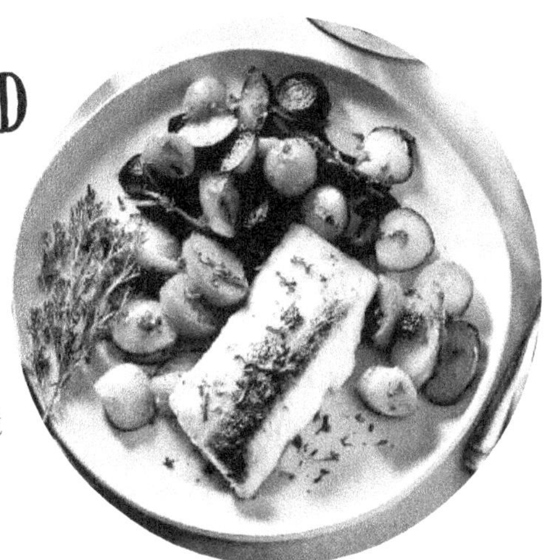

Servings: 4 | Prep Time: 15 minutes | Cook Time: 25 minutes | Carbs per Serving: 10g

INGREDIENTS

- 4 cod fillets
- 2 cups mixed vegetables (zucchini, bell peppers, carrots)
- 2 tbsp olive oil
- 1 tsp dried thyme
- 1 tsp dried rosemary
- 1 tsp paprika
- Salt and pepper to taste
- Lemon wedges for serving

DIRECTIONS

1. Preheat oven to 400°F (200°C).
2. Toss mixed vegetables with olive oil, dried thyme, dried rosemary, paprika, salt, and pepper.
3. Spread vegetables on a baking sheet and roast in the oven for 20-25 minutes until tender.
4. Season cod fillets with salt and pepper.
5. Place cod fillets on another baking sheet lined with parchment paper.
6. Bake cod in the oven for 12-15 minutes or until fish flakes easily with a fork.
7. Serve baked cod with roasted vegetables and lemon wedges.

NUTRIENT CONTENT (PER SERVING):

- Calories: 280
- Total Fat: 12g
- Protein: 30g
- Carbohydrates: 10g
- Sugars: 4g
- Fiber: 3g
- Sodium: 320mg

INGREDIENT TIPS:

- Cod Fillets: Lean white fish that's low in calories and high in protein, perfect for blood sugar control.
- Mixed Vegetables: Colorful assortment of veggies adds vitamins, minerals, and fiber to the dish.
- Herbs and Spices: Dried thyme, rosemary, and paprika enhance the flavors without extra calories or sodium.

LEMON GARLIC HERB GRILLED SHRIMP

This Lemon Garlic Herb Grilled Shrimp is a light and flavorful dish that's quick to prepare and perfect for a healthy meal. The combination of grilled shrimp with zesty lemon, garlic, and fresh herbs creates a delightful culinary experience.

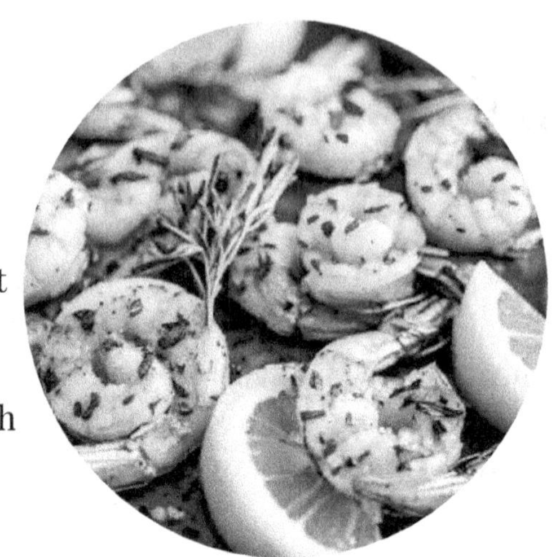

Servings: 4 | Prep Time: 15 minutes | Cook Time: 6 minutes | Carbs per Serving: 2g

INGREDIENTS

- 1 lb large shrimp, peeled and deveined
- 2 tbsp olive oil
- 2 cloves garlic, minced
- Zest and juice of 1 lemon
- 1 tbsp chopped fresh parsley
- 1 tsp dried oregano
- Salt and pepper to taste
- Skewers (if using wooden, soak in water for 30 minutes)

DIRECTIONS

1. In a bowl, whisk together olive oil, minced garlic, lemon zest, lemon juice, chopped parsley, dried oregano, salt, and pepper to make the marinade.
2. Add shrimp to the marinade and toss to coat evenly. Let marinate for 15-30 minutes.
3. Preheat grill to medium-high heat.
4. Thread shrimp onto skewers.
5. Grill shrimp skewers for 2-3 minutes per side or until shrimp are pink and cooked through.
6. Remove from grill and serve hot.

NUTRIENT CONTENT (PER SERVING):

- Calories: 180
- Total Fat: 8g
- Protein: 25g
- Carbohydrates: 2g
- Sugars: 0g
- Fiber: 0g
- Sodium: 320mg

INGREDIENT TIPS:

- Large Shrimp: Low in calories and high in protein, shrimp is a versatile seafood option.
- Lemon and Garlic: Provide flavor without added sugars or carbs, enhancing the taste of grilled shrimp.

BAKED LEMON HERB TILAPIA

This Baked Lemon Herb Tilapia is a light and nutritious dish that's perfect for a healthy dinner option. Tilapia is a mild-flavored fish that pairs well with zesty lemon and herbs, creating a delicious and diabetes-friendly meal.

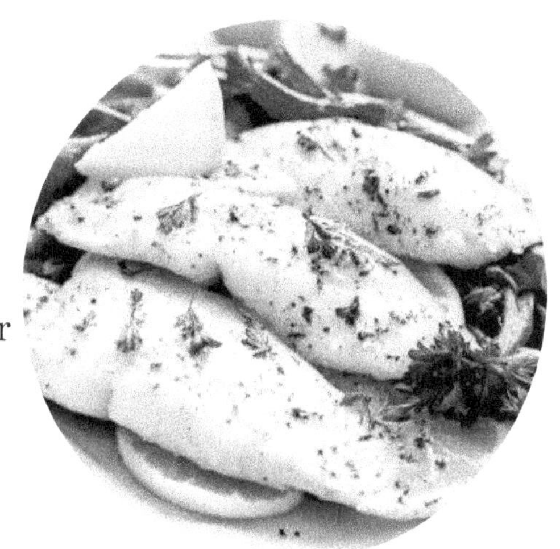

Servings: 4 | Prep Time: 10 minutes | Cook Time: 15 minutes | Carbs per Serving: 2g

INGREDIENTS

- 4 tilapia fillets
- 2 tbsp olive oil
- Zest and juice of 1 lemon
- 1 tsp dried thyme
- 1 tsp dried rosemary
- Salt and pepper to taste
- Lemon slices for serving
- Fresh parsley for garnish

DIRECTIONS

1. Preheat oven to 375°F (190°C).
2. Place tilapia fillets on a baking sheet lined with parchment paper.
3. In a bowl, combine olive oil, lemon zest, lemon juice, dried thyme, dried rosemary, salt, and pepper to make the marinade.
4. Brush the marinade over the tilapia fillets, coating them evenly.
5. Bake tilapia in the preheated oven for 12–15 minutes or until fish is cooked through and flakes easily with a fork.
6. Serve baked tilapia hot, garnished with lemon slices and fresh parsley.

NUTRIENT CONTENT (PER SERVING):

- Calories: 150
- Total Fat: 7g
- Protein: 20g
- Carbohydrates: 2g
- Sugars: 0g
- Fiber: 0g
- Sodium: 300mg

INGREDIENT TIPS:

- Tilapia Fillets: Mild-flavored white fish that's low in calories and rich in protein.
- Lemon and Herbs: Add flavor without added sugars or carbs, enhancing the taste of baked tilapia.

Chapter Ten

SAUCE, DIPS, & DRESSINGS

This chapter is dedicated to providing you with versatile and delicious condiments that not only enhance the taste of your meals but also support your journey towards stable blood sugar levels and overall well-being.

Sauces, dips, and dressings are often the secret ingredients that turn ordinary meals into extraordinary culinary experiences. However, when managing pre-diabetes, it's essential to choose options that are low in added sugars, saturated fats, and unnecessary calories. That's why the recipes in this chapter are thoughtfully crafted to be diabetes-friendly while still delivering on taste and texture.

From tangy vinaigrettes and creamy dips to savory sauces and marinades, each recipe is designed to complement a wide range of dishes, including meats, salads, vegetables, and more. By incorporating these homemade condiments into your cooking routine, you'll have the freedom to create flavorful meals while keeping your blood sugar levels in check.

Whether you're looking to add a burst of flavor to grilled proteins, elevate the taste of your salads, or enjoy guilt-free dips with your snacks, this chapter has something for every palate. Let's explore the world of sauces, dips, and dressings that make your pre-diabetic diet both satisfying and delicious.

SPICY SRIRACHA MAYO

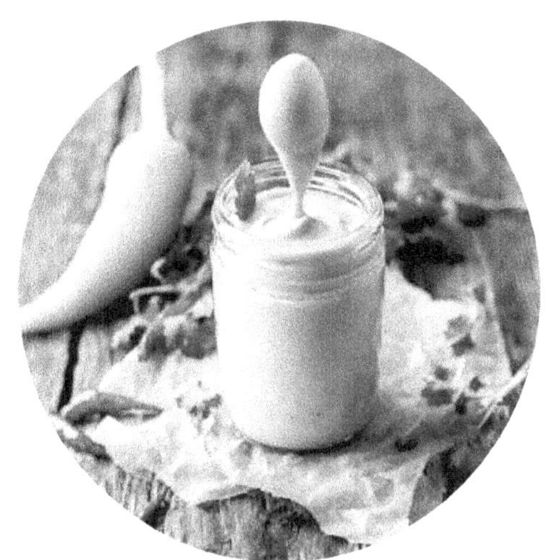

Spicy and zesty Sriracha mayo, perfect for adding a kick to your favorite dishes.

Servings: 8 | Prep Time: 5 mins | Carbs per Serving: 2g

INGREDIENTS

- 1/2 cup mayonnaise
- 2 tablespoons Sriracha sauce (adjust to taste for spiciness)
- 1 tablespoon lime juice
- 1 teaspoon honey or maple syrup (optional, for sweetness)
- Salt to taste

DIRECTIONS

1. In a bowl, combine mayonnaise, Sriracha sauce, lime juice, and honey or maple syrup (if using).
2. Mix well until all ingredients are thoroughly combined.
3. Taste and adjust the spiciness with more Sriracha or balance with honey/maple syrup.
4. Add salt to taste.
5. Transfer the spicy Sriracha mayo to a serving bowl or squeeze bottle.
6. Use as a dip for fries, chicken tenders, or as a spread for sandwiches and burgers.

NUTRIENT CONTENT (PER SERVING):		INGREDIENT TIPS:
• Calories: 90 • Total Fat: 10g • Protein: 0g • Carbohydrates: 2g	• Sugars: 1g • Fiber: 0g • Sodium: 130mg	Sriracha adds heat and flavor, while lime juice provides tanginess. Adjust sweetness and spiciness to suit your preference.

CREAMY GARLIC PARMESAN DIP

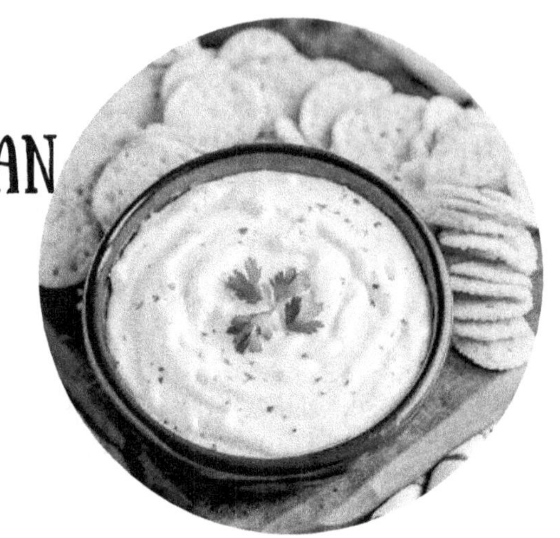

Creamy and flavorful garlic Parmesan dip, perfect for dunking your favorite snacks or adding a burst of flavor to meals.

Servings: 8 | Prep Time: 10 mins | Chill Time: 30 mins | Carbs per Serving: 3g

INGREDIENTS

- 1 cup sour cream
- 1/2 cup grated Parmesan cheese
- 2 cloves garlic, minced
- 1 tablespoon fresh parsley, chopped
- 1 tablespoon lemon juice
- Salt and pepper to taste

DIRECTIONS

1. In a bowl, combine sour cream, grated Parmesan cheese, minced garlic, chopped parsley, and lemon juice.
2. Mix until the ingredients are well incorporated and the dip is creamy.
3. Season with salt and pepper to taste.
4. Cover and refrigerate the creamy garlic Parmesan dip for at least 30 minutes before serving.
5. Garnish with additional parsley before serving, if desired.
6. Serve as a dip for veggies, chips, or as a topping for baked potatoes.

NUTRIENT CONTENT (PER SERVING):		INGREDIENT TIPS:
• Calories: 120 • Total Fat: 10g • Protein: 3g • Carbohydrates: 3g	• Sugars: 1g • Fiber: 0g • Sodium: 150mg	Fresh garlic and Parmesan cheese provide bold flavors, while lemon juice adds brightness. Adjust seasoning to your liking.

AVOCADO LIME DRESSING

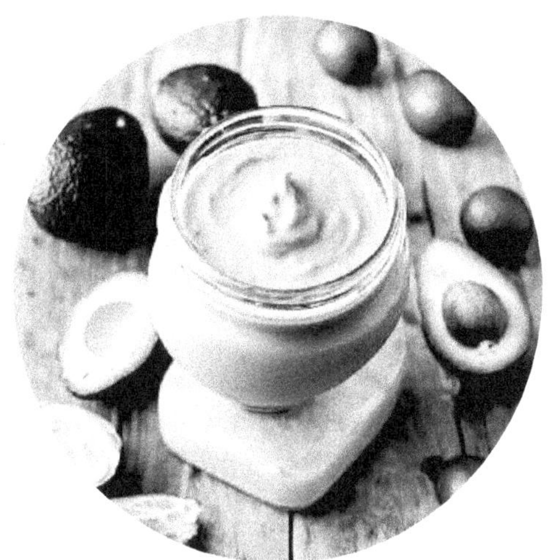

Creamy and zesty avocado lime dressing, perfect for adding a burst of flavor to your salads and meals.

Servings: 8 | Prep Time: 10 mins | Carbs per Serving: 3g

INGREDIENTS

- 1 ripe avocado, peeled and pitted
- 1/4 cup plain Greek yogurt
- Juice of 1 lime
- 2 tablespoons fresh cilantro, chopped
- 1 clove garlic, minced
- 2 tablespoons extra virgin olive oil
- Salt and pepper to taste
- Water (as needed for desired consistency)

DIRECTIONS

1. In a blender or food processor, combine the avocado, Greek yogurt, lime juice, chopped cilantro, minced garlic, olive oil, salt, and pepper.
2. Blend until smooth and creamy.
3. If the dressing is too thick, add water a little at a time until you reach your desired consistency.
4. Taste and adjust seasoning as needed.
5. Transfer the avocado lime dressing to a jar or container with a tight lid.
6. Refrigerate until ready to use.
7. Serve drizzled over salads, as a dip for veggies, or as a sauce for grilled chicken or fish.

NUTRIENT CONTENT (PER SERVING):		INGREDIENT TIPS:
• Calories: 80 • Total Fat: 7g • Protein: 2g • Carbohydrates: 3g	• Sugars: 0g • Fiber: 2g • Sodium: 40mg	Avocado provides creaminess and healthy fats, while lime juice and cilantro add refreshing flavor. Adjust garlic and seasoning to your taste.

TANGY HONEY MUSTARD DIP

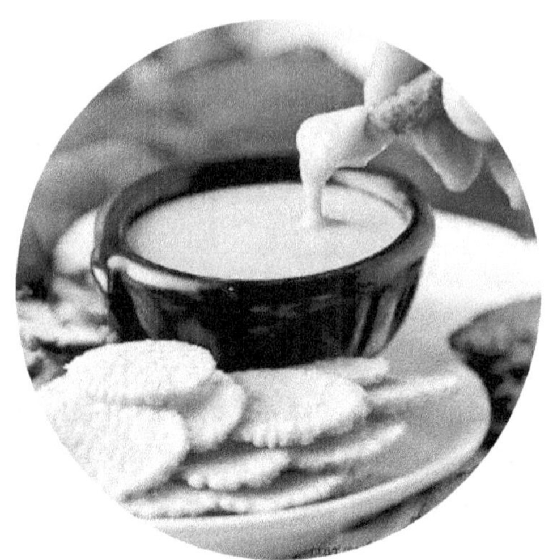

Tangy and sweet honey mustard dip, perfect for dipping or as a flavorful sauce for a variety of dishes.

Servings: 8 | Prep Time: 5 mins | Chill Time: 30 mins | Carbs per Serving: 5g

INGREDIENTS

- 1/2 cup mayonnaise
- 2 tablespoons Dijon mustard
- 2 tablespoons honey
- 1 tablespoon apple cider vinegar
- 1 clove garlic, minced
- Salt and pepper to taste

DIRECTIONS

1. In a bowl, whisk together mayonnaise, Dijon mustard, honey, apple cider vinegar, minced garlic, salt, and pepper until well combined.
2. Taste and adjust the sweetness and tanginess by adding more honey or vinegar as needed.
3. Season with salt and pepper to taste.
4. Transfer the tangy honey mustard dip to a serving bowl.
5. Chill in the refrigerator for at least 30 minutes before serving to allow flavors to meld.
6. Serve as a dip for chicken tenders, pretzels, or as a sauce for sandwiches and wraps.

NUTRIENT CONTENT (PER SERVING):		INGREDIENT TIPS:
• Calories: 120 • Total Fat: 10g • Protein: 0g • Carbohydrates: 5g	• Sugars: 5g • Fiber: 0g • Sodium: 130mg	The combination of Dijon mustard, honey, and vinegar creates a balance of sweet, tangy, and savory flavors. Adjust ingredients to achieve your preferred taste.

LEMON HERB YOGURT SAUCE

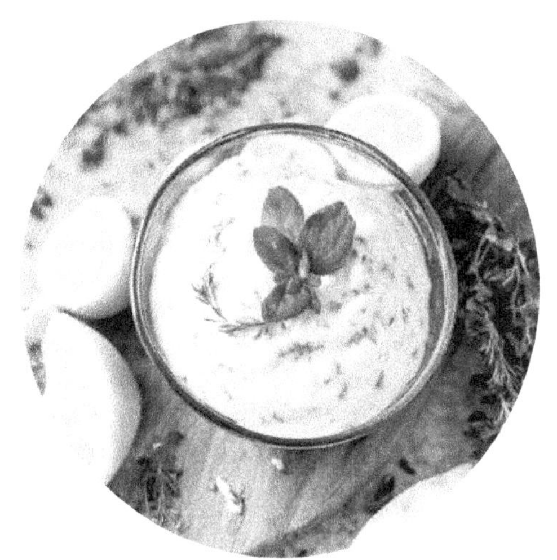

Refreshing and zesty lemon herb yogurt sauce, perfect for adding a burst of flavor to your dishes.

Servings: 8 | Prep Time: 10 mins | Chill Time: 30 mins | Carbs per Serving: 3g

INGREDIENTS

- 1 cup plain Greek yogurt
- Zest and juice of 1 lemon
- 2 tablespoons fresh parsley, chopped
- 1 tablespoon fresh dill, chopped
- 1 clove garlic, minced
- Salt and pepper to taste

DIRECTIONS

1. In a bowl, combine Greek yogurt, lemon zest, lemon juice, chopped parsley, chopped dill, minced garlic, salt, and pepper.
2. Mix well until all ingredients are evenly incorporated.
3. Taste and adjust seasoning as needed, adding more lemon juice for tanginess or herbs for flavor.
4. Refrigerate the lemon herb yogurt sauce for at least 30 minutes before serving to allow the flavors to meld.
5. Stir again before serving.
6. Use as a sauce for grilled chicken, fish, or roasted vegetables, or as a dip for fresh veggies and pita chips.

NUTRIENT CONTENT (PER SERVING):

- Calories: 50
- Total Fat: 0g
- Protein: 6g
- Carbohydrates: 3g
- Sugars: 2g
- Fiber: 0g
- Sodium: 25mg

INGREDIENT TIPS:

Fresh lemon and herbs add brightness and freshness to the creamy yogurt base. Customize with your favorite herbs for variations.

CREAMY CILANTRO LIME DRESSING

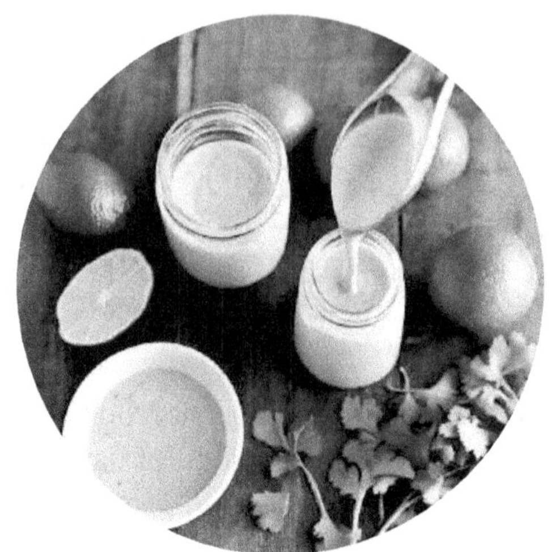

Creamy and tangy cilantro lime dressing, perfect for adding a zesty kick to your favorite salads and dishes.

Servings: 8 | Prep Time: 10 mins | Chill Time: 1 hour | Carbs per Serving: 3g

INGREDIENTS

- 1/2 cup mayonnaise
- 1/4 cup sour cream
- 2 tablespoons fresh cilantro, chopped
- Juice of 1 lime
- 1 clove garlic, minced
- 1 teaspoon honey
- Salt and pepper to taste

DIRECTIONS

1. In a bowl, combine mayonnaise, sour cream, chopped cilantro, lime juice, minced garlic, honey, salt, and pepper.
2. Whisk until the ingredients are well combined and the dressing is smooth.
3. Taste and adjust seasoning, adding more lime juice for tanginess or honey for sweetness.
4. Refrigerate the creamy cilantro lime dressing for at least 1 hour before serving to allow the flavors to meld.
5. Stir again before using.
6. Serve as a dressing for salads, drizzle over grilled meats or seafood, or use as a dip for tacos and wraps.

NUTRIENT CONTENT (PER SERVING):		INGREDIENT TIPS:
• Calories: 120 • Total Fat: 12g • Protein: 1g • Carbohydrates: 3g	• Sugars: 2g • Fiber: 0g • Sodium: 100mg	The combination of cilantro, lime, and honey creates a creamy and flavorful dressing with a hint of sweetness. Adjust ingredients to your taste preferences.

AVOCADO YOGURT DIP

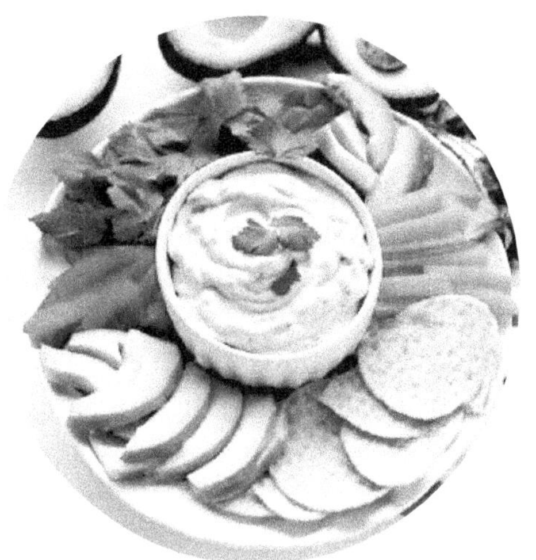

This Avocado Yogurt Dip is a creamy and nutritious option for pairing with raw veggies or whole-grain crackers. Avocado provides healthy fats, while yogurt adds protein and probiotics, making it a diabetes-friendly choice.

Servings: 6 | Prep Time: 10 minutes | Carbs per Serving: 4g | Calories: 70

INGREDIENTS

- 1 ripe avocado
- 1/2 cup plain Greek yogurt
- 1 clove garlic, minced
- 2 tbsp fresh lemon juice
- 1 tbsp chopped fresh cilantro
- Salt and pepper to taste

DIRECTIONS

1. Scoop the flesh of the ripe avocado into a bowl.
2. Add Greek yogurt, minced garlic, lemon juice, chopped cilantro, salt, and pepper to the bowl.
3. Mash and mix the ingredients together until smooth and well combined.
4. Adjust seasoning to taste.
5. Serve the avocado yogurt dip with vegetable sticks or whole-grain crackers.

NUTRIENT CONTENT (PER SERVING):	INGREDIENT TIPS:
• Calories: 70 • Total Fat: 5g • Protein: 3g • Carbohydrates: 4g • Sugars: 0g • Fiber: 3g • Sodium: 15mg	• Avocado: Provides healthy monounsaturated fats and fiber, contributing to satiety and heart health. • Greek Yogurt: Adds protein, probiotics, and creaminess to the dip without excessive sugars.

TANGY BALSAMIC VINAIGRETTE

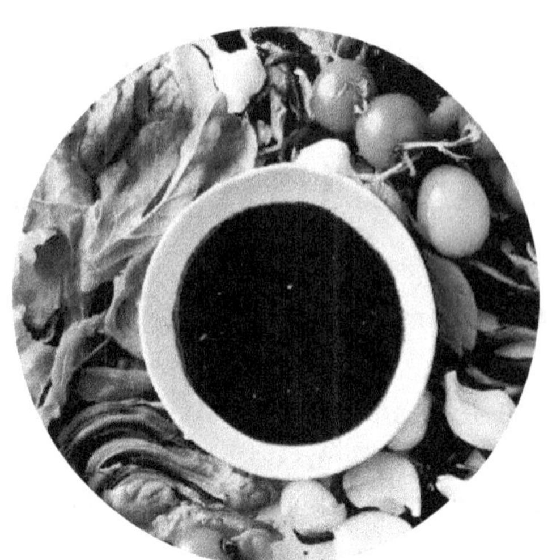

This Tangy Balsamic Vinaigrette is a flavorful dressing for salads and grilled vegetables. With a perfect balance of tanginess and sweetness, it enhances your dishes while keeping blood sugar levels stable.

Servings: 6 | Prep Time: 5 minutes | Carbs per Serving: 2g | Calories: 50

INGREDIENTS

- 1/4 cup balsamic vinegar
- 2 tbsp extra virgin olive oil
- 1 tsp Dijon mustard
- 1 tsp honey or agave syrup (optional for sweetness)
- 1 clove garlic, minced
- Salt and pepper to taste

DIRECTIONS

1. In a small bowl, whisk together balsamic vinegar, olive oil, Dijon mustard, minced garlic, honey or agave syrup (if using), salt, and pepper until well combined.
2. Adjust sweetness and seasoning to taste.
3. Use the tangy balsamic vinaigrette as a dressing for salads or marinade for grilled vegetables.

NUTRIENT CONTENT (PER SERVING):	INGREDIENT TIPS:
• Calories: 50 • Total Fat: 4g • Protein: 0g • Carbohydrates: 2g • Sugars: 1g • Fiber: 0g • Sodium: 60mg	• Balsamic Vinegar: Adds flavor without added sugars, perfect for a diabetes-friendly dressing. • Extra Virgin Olive Oil: Provides heart-healthy fats and richness to the vinaigrette

ROASTED RED PEPPER HUMMUS

This Roasted Red Pepper Hummus is a delicious and fiber-rich dip that pairs well with whole-grain pita bread or vegetable sticks. Chickpeas, the main ingredient, are a good source of protein and complex carbs, ideal for managing blood sugar levels.

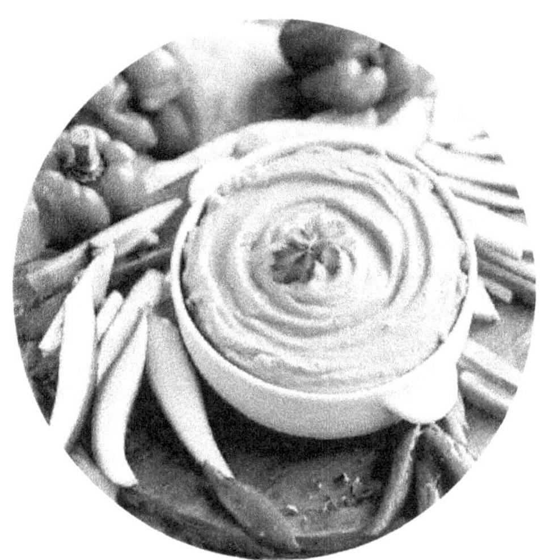

Servings: 8 | Prep Time: 10 minutes | Carbs per Serving: 5g | Calories: 70

INGREDIENTS

- 1 can (15 oz) chickpeas, drained and rinsed
- 1/4 cup roasted red peppers (from jar or homemade)
- 2 tbsp tahini
- 2 tbsp lemon juice
- 1 clove garlic, minced
- 2 tbsp extra virgin olive oil
- Salt and cumin to taste
- Water (as needed for consistency)

DIRECTIONS

1. In a food processor, combine chickpeas, roasted red peppers, tahini, lemon juice, minced garlic, olive oil, salt, and cumin.
2. Blend until smooth, adding water as needed to achieve desired consistency.
3. Taste and adjust seasoning if necessary.
4. Transfer the roasted red pepper hummus to a serving bowl.
5. Drizzle with a little extra olive oil and sprinkle with cumin before serving.

NUTRIENT CONTENT (PER SERVING):

- Calories: 70
- Total Fat: 4g
- Protein: 2g
- Carbohydrates: 5g
- Sugars: 0g
- Fiber: 1g
- Sodium: 120mg

INGREDIENT TIPS:

- Chickpeas: Provide protein, fiber, and complex carbs, promoting satiety and stable blood sugar levels.
- Roasted Red Peppers: Add flavor and color to the hummus without added sugars.

Chapter Eleven

Smoothies

Smoothies are an excellent way to incorporate a variety of healthy ingredients into your diet in a convenient and enjoyable manner. They offer a perfect blend of fruits, vegetables, proteins, and healthy fats, making them ideal for a balanced and diabetes-friendly diet.

This chapter is dedicated to providing you with delicious and nutrient-packed smoothie recipes that not only tantalize your taste buds but also support your journey towards stable blood sugar levels and overall well-being. In the chapter, you'll discover a collection of smoothie recipes that are low in added sugars, high in fiber, and packed with essential vitamins and minerals. Each recipe is carefully crafted to help you manage blood sugar spikes, promote satiety, and provide a refreshing and nourishing treat.

Whether you're looking for a quick breakfast option, a post-workout refresher, or a satisfying snack, these smoothies are designed to be both delicious and supportive of your pre-diabetic dietary needs. Let's dive into the world of flavorful and nutritious smoothies that make your wellness journey both enjoyable and beneficial.

BERRY BLISS DELIGHT

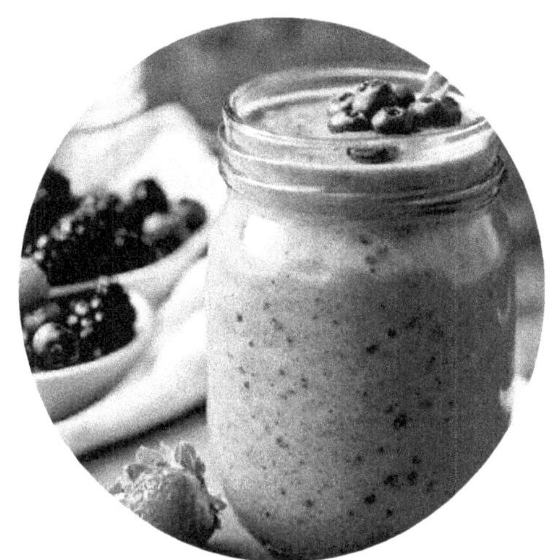

This smoothie combines mixed berries' antioxidant-rich goodness with Greek yogurt's creaminess and the nourishing benefits of chia seeds and almond butter.

Servings: 1 | Prep Time: 5 minutes | Cook Time: 0 minutes | Carbs per Serving: 20g

INGREDIENTS

- 1/2 cup mixed berries (such as strawberries, blueberries, and raspberries)
- 1/2 cup plain Greek yogurt
- 1 tablespoon chia seeds
- 1 tablespoon almond butter
- 1 teaspoon honey (optional)
- 1 cup unsweetened almond milk

DIRECTIONS

1. Combine mixed berries, Greek yogurt, chia seeds, almond butter, honey (if using), and almond milk in a blender.
2. Blend until smooth and creamy.
3. Pour into a glass and savor the delightful blend of berries and nutritious ingredients.

NUTRIENT CONTENT (PER SERVING):

- Calories: 250
- Total Fat: 12g
- Protein: 15g
- Carbohydrates: 20g
- Sugars: 12g
- Fiber: 6g
- Sodium: 100mg

HELPFUL INFO:

The Berry Bliss Delight smoothie is a tasty treat that supports glucose balance and satisfies your taste buds.

TROPICAL TURMERIC DELIGHT

A smoothie that combines the exotic flavors of pineapple, mango, and turmeric, complemented by the richness of coconut oil and hemp seeds.

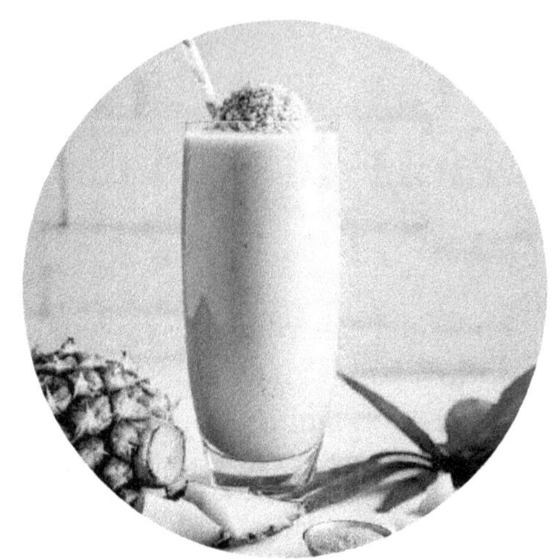

Servings: 1 | Prep Time: 5 minutes | Cook Time: 0 minutes | Carbs per Serving: 30g

INGREDIENTS

- 1/2 cup pineapple chunks (fresh or frozen)
- 1/2 cup mango chunks (fresh or frozen)
- 1/2 inch fresh turmeric root (or 1/2 teaspoon ground turmeric)
- 1 tablespoon coconut oil
- 1 tablespoon hemp seeds
- 1 cup coconut water

DIRECTIONS

1. Add pineapple chunks, mango chunks, fresh turmeric root (or ground turmeric), coconut oil, hemp seeds, and coconut water to a blender.
2. Blend until smooth and creamy.
3. Pour into a glass and enjoy the tropical flavors with the added benefits of turmeric and coconut.

NUTRIENT CONTENT (PER SERVING):		HELPFUL INFO:
• Calories: 300 • Total Fat: 15g • Protein: 5g • Carbohydrates: 30g	• Sugars: 20g • Fiber: 6g • Sodium: 50mg	This vibrant smoothie delights your taste buds and supports balanced blood sugar levels and overall wellness.

SPINACH BERRY BLAST

The Spinach Berry Blast smoothie combines the power of leafy greens with the sweetness of mixed berries and the richness of almond butter and flaxseed meal.

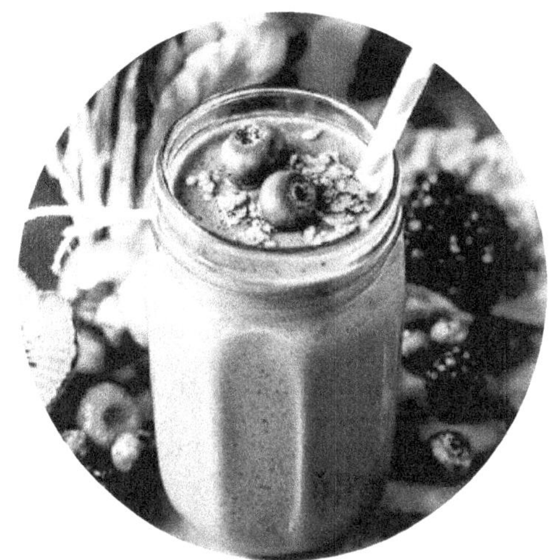

Servings: 1 | Prep Time: 5 minutes | Cook Time: 0 minutes | Carbs per Serving: 25g

INGREDIENTS

- 1 cup fresh spinach leaves
- 1/2 cup mixed berries (such as strawberries, blueberries, and blackberries)
- 1/2 banana
- 1 tablespoon almond butter
- 1 tablespoon flaxseed meal
- 1 cup unsweetened almond milk

DIRECTIONS

1. Place fresh spinach leaves, mixed berries, banana, almond butter, flaxseed meal, and almond milk in a blender.
2. Blend until smooth and creamy.
3. Pour into a glass and enjoy the nutritious goodness of leafy greens and berries.

NUTRIENT CONTENT (PER SERVING):

- Calories: 230
- Total Fat: 11g
- Protein: 7g
- Carbohydrates: 25g
- Sugars: 10g
- Fiber: 8g
- Sodium: 120mg

HELPFUL INFO:

This refreshing smoothie is packed with vitamins, antioxidants, and fiber to support glucose balance and overall health for women over 50.

CINNAMON APPLE PIE DELIGHT

A smoothie that captures the essence of a classic dessert with the wholesome goodness of apples, cinnamon, almond butter, chai seeds and nutmeg.

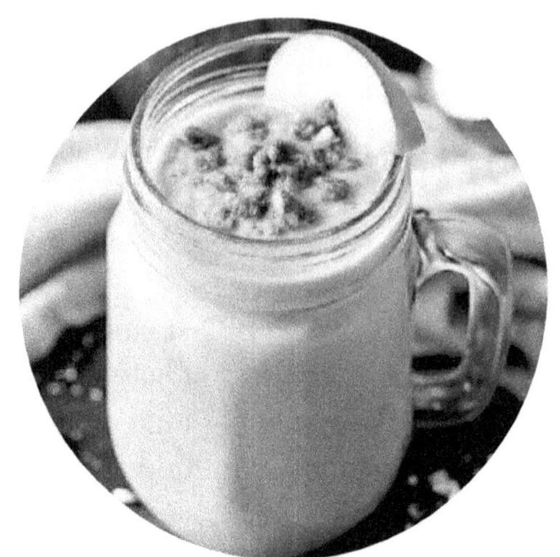

Servings: 1 | Prep Time: 5 minutes | Cook Time: 0 minutes | Carbs per Serving: 20g

INGREDIENTS

- 1 medium apple, cored and sliced
- 1/2 teaspoon ground cinnamon
- 1/4 teaspoon nutmeg
- 1 tablespoon almond butter
- 1 tablespoon chia seeds
- 1 cup unsweetened almond milk

DIRECTIONS

1. Place apple slices, ground cinnamon, nutmeg, almond butter, chia seeds, and almond milk in a blender.
2. Blend until smooth and creamy.
3. Pour into a glass and savor the comforting flavors of apple pie in a healthy smoothie form.

NUTRIENT CONTENT (PER SERVING):		HELPFUL INFO:
• Calories: 220 • Total Fat: 10g • Protein: 5g • Carbohydrates: 20g	• Sugars: 10g • Fiber: 8g • Sodium: 100mg	With the added benefits of almond butter and chia seeds, this smoothie is a delightful treat that supports blood sugar balance and satisfies your taste buds.

BERRY AVOCADO POWERHOUSE

A smoothie that combines the antioxidant-rich berries with the creamy texture of avocado boosted by Greek yogurt and pumpkin seeds.

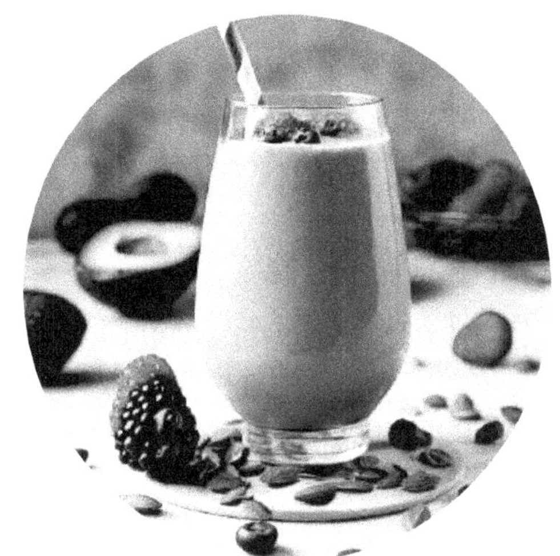

Servings: 1　|　Prep Time: 5 minutes　|　Cook Time: 0 minutes　|　Carbs per Serving: 15g

INGREDIENTS

- 1/2 cup mixed berries (such as raspberries, strawberries, and blueberries)
- 1/4 avocado, peeled and pitted
- 1 tablespoon Greek yogurt
- 1 tablespoon pumpkin seeds
- 1 teaspoon honey (optional)
- 1 cup coconut water

DIRECTIONS

1. Combine mixed berries, avocado, Greek yogurt, pumpkin seeds, honey (if using), and coconut water in a blender.
2. Blend until smooth and creamy.
3. Pour into a glass and enjoy the nutrient-packed goodness of berries and avocado.

NUTRIENT CONTENT (PER SERVING):		HELPFUL INFO:
• Calories: 250 • Total Fat: 15g • Protein: 6g • Carbohydrates: 15g	• Sugars: 8g • Fiber: 6g • Sodium: 80mg	This powerhouse smoothie provides essential nutrients and healthy fats, promoting glucose balance and overall vitality for women over 50.

TROPICAL MANGO TANGO

A refreshing blend of tropical fruits like mango and pineapple, complemented by the warmth of ginger and the nutritional boost of flaxseeds.

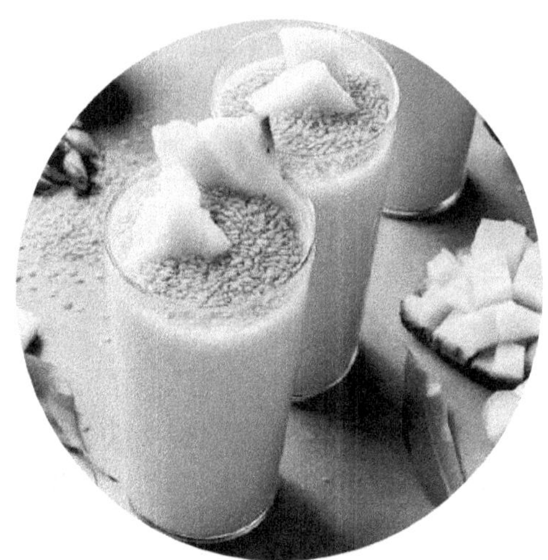

Servings: 1 | Prep Time: 5 minutes | Cook Time: 0 minutes | Carbs per Serving: 25g

INGREDIENTS

- 1/2 cup frozen mango chunks
- 1/4 cup pineapple chunks
- 1/4 cup Greek yogurt
- 1 tablespoon flaxseeds
- 1 teaspoon grated ginger
- 1 cup coconut milk (unsweetened)

DIRECTIONS

1. Combine frozen mango chunks, pineapple chunks, Greek yogurt, flaxseeds, grated ginger, and coconut milk in a blender.
2. Blend until smooth and creamy.
3. Pour into a glass and enjoy the tropical flavors of mango and pineapple with a hint of ginger.

NUTRIENT CONTENT (PER SERVING):		HELPFUL INFO:
• Calories: 280 • Total Fat: 12g • Protein: 7g • Carbohydrates: 25g	• Sugars: 18g • Fiber: 5g • Sodium: 90mg	The Tropical Mango Tango smoothie contains vitamins, fiber, and healthy fats. This smoothie is a delicious way to support glucose balance and satisfy your taste buds.

CHOCOLATE PEANUT BUTTER BLISS

A dreamy smoothie combination of chocolate, peanut butter, and banana, elevated with the nutritious addition of hemp seeds.

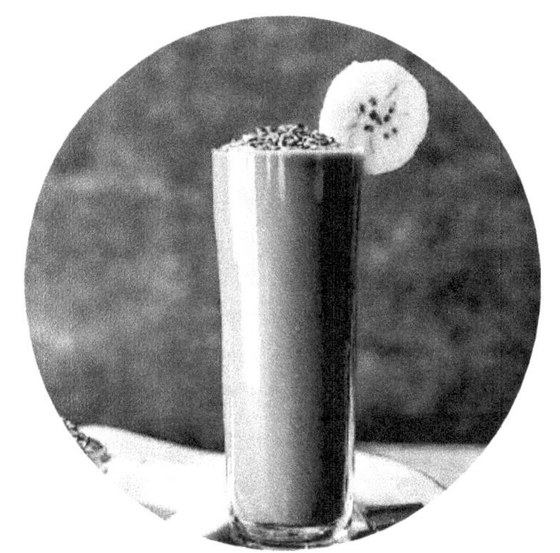

Servings: 1 | Prep Time: 5 minutes | Cook Time: 0 minutes | Carbs per Serving: 30g

INGREDIENTS

- 1 ripe banana
- 1 tablespoon unsweetened cocoa powder
- 1 tablespoon natural peanut butter
- 1 tablespoon hemp seeds
- 1 cup almond milk (unsweetened)
- Ice cubes (optional)

DIRECTIONS

1. In a blender, combine the ripe banana, cocoa powder, natural peanut butter, hemp seeds, almond milk, and ice cubes if desired.
2. Blend until smooth and creamy.
3. Pour into a glass and indulge in the rich, chocolatey goodness of this smoothie.

NUTRIENT CONTENT (PER SERVING):

- Calories: 300
- Total Fat: 14g
- Protein: 8g
- Carbohydrates: 30g
- Sugars: 15g
- Fiber: 6g
- Sodium: 120mg

HELPFUL INFO:

The Chocolate Peanut Butter Bliss smoothie is a decadent yet wholesome smoothie. Perfect for satisfying cravings while supporting balanced blood sugar levels.

GREEN POWER SMOOTHIE

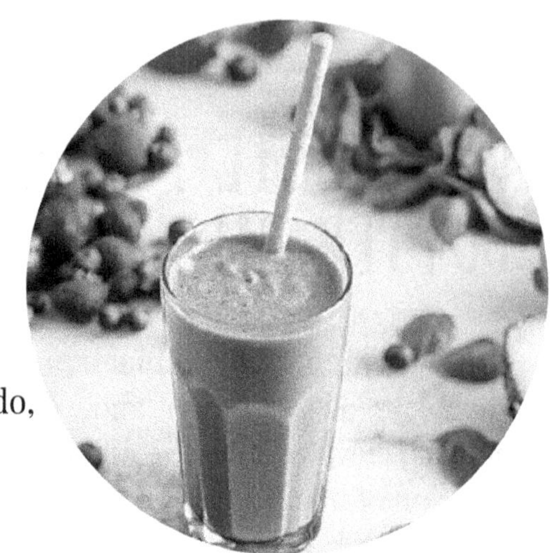

This Green Power Smoothie is packed with nutrient-rich ingredients like spinach, avocado, and Greek yogurt, making it a satisfying and diabetes-friendly breakfast option or snack.

Servings: 1 | Prep Time: 5 minutes | Carbs per Serving: 15g | Calories: 250

INGREDIENTS

- 1 cup fresh spinach leaves
- 1/2 ripe avocado
- 1/2 cup Greek yogurt
- 1/2 cup unsweetened almond milk
- 1 tbsp chia seeds
- 1/2 banana (optional for sweetness)
- Ice cubes (optional)
- Stevia or honey (optional for added sweetness)

DIRECTIONS

1. In a blender, combine spinach, avocado, Greek yogurt, almond milk, chia seeds, banana (if using), and ice cubes.
2. Blend until smooth and creamy.
3. Taste and sweeten with stevia or honey if desired.
4. Pour into a glass and enjoy immediately.

NUTRIENT CONTENT (PER SERVING):

- Calories: 250
- Total Fat: 15g
- Protein: 10g
- Carbohydrates: 15g
- Sugars: 5g
- Fiber: 7g
- Sodium: 120mg

HELPFUL INFO:

- Spinach: Rich in vitamins, minerals, and fiber, spinach adds nutritional value without spiking blood sugar levels.
- Avocado: Provides healthy fats and creaminess to the smoothie, enhancing satiety and texture.
- Chia Seeds: High in fiber and omega-3 fatty acids, chia seeds promote digestive health and heart health.

BERRY BLAST SMOOTHIE

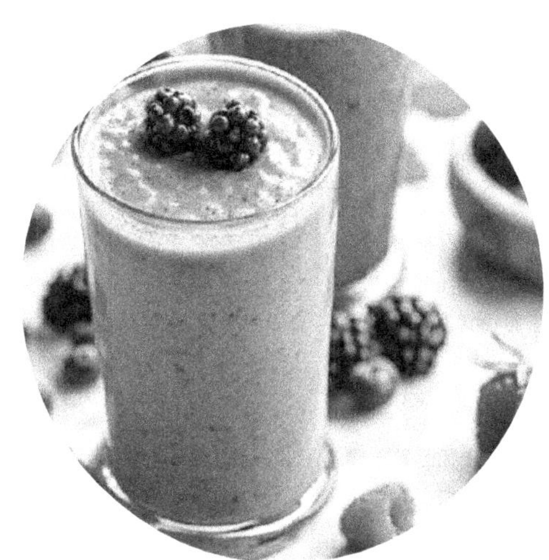

This Berry Blast Smoothie combines antioxidant-rich berries with protein-packed Greek yogurt for a delicious and blood sugar-friendly treat.

Servings: 1 | Prep Time: 5 minutes | Carbs per Serving: 15g | Calories: 200

INGREDIENTS

- 1/2 cup mixed berries (strawberries, blueberries, raspberries)
- 1/2 cup Greek yogurt
- 1/2 cup unsweetened almond milk
- 1 tbsp flaxseed meal
- 1/2 tsp vanilla extract
- Ice cubes (optional)
- Stevia or honey (optional for added sweetness)

DIRECTIONS

1. In a blender, combine mixed berries, Greek yogurt, almond milk, flaxseed meal, vanilla extract, and ice cubes.
2. Blend until smooth and well combined.
3. Taste and sweeten with stevia or honey if desired.
4. Pour into a glass and serve immediately.

NUTRIENT CONTENT (PER SERVING):

- Calories: 200
- Total Fat: 8g
- Protein: 12g
- Carbohydrates: 15g
- Sugars: 8g
- Fiber: 5g
- Sodium: 120mg

HELPFUL INFO:

- Mixed Berries: Packed with antioxidants and fiber, berries add sweetness and nutritional benefits to the smoothie.
- Greek Yogurt: High in protein and probiotics, Greek yogurt supports gut health and provides satiety.
- Flaxseed Meal: Adds omega-3 fatty acids and fiber, promoting heart health and digestive health.

TROPICAL PARADISE SMOOTHIE

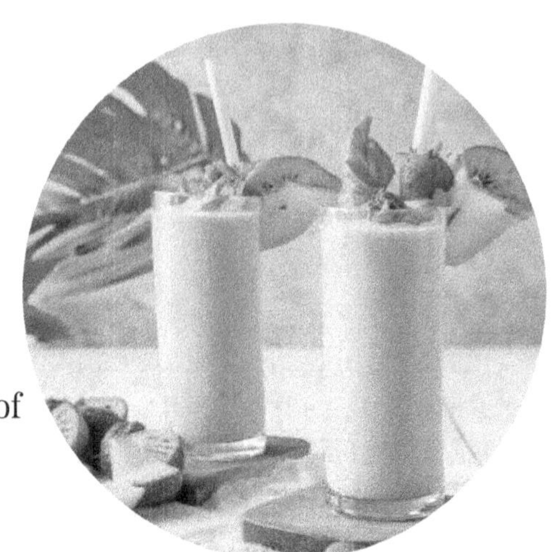

This Tropical Paradise Smoothie combines tropical fruits with coconut milk and a touch of ginger for a refreshing and diabetes-friendly beverage.

Servings: 1 | Prep Time: 5 minutes | Carbs per Serving: 30g |

INGREDIENTS

- 1/2 cup pineapple chunks
- 1/2 banana
- 1/2 cup mango chunks
- 1/2 cup coconut milk (unsweetened)
- 1 tsp grated fresh ginger
- Ice cubes (optional)
- Stevia or honey (optional for added sweetness)

DIRECTIONS

1. In a blender, combine pineapple chunks, banana, mango chunks, coconut milk, grated ginger, and ice cubes.
2. Blend until smooth and creamy.
3. Taste and sweeten with stevia or honey if desired.
4. Pour into a glass and enjoy immediately.

NUTRIENT CONTENT (PER SERVING):

- Calories: 250
- Total Fat: 10g
- Protein: 3g
- Carbohydrates: 30g
- Sugars: 20g
- Fiber: 5g
- Sodium: 30mg

HELPFUL INFO:

- Tropical Fruits: Pineapple, banana, and mango are rich in vitamins, minerals, and fiber, adding sweetness and tropical flavor to the smoothie.
- Coconut Milk: Provides healthy fats and a creamy texture without added sugars, perfect for a diabetes-friendly beverage.

ALMOND BUTTER BANANA SMOOTHIE

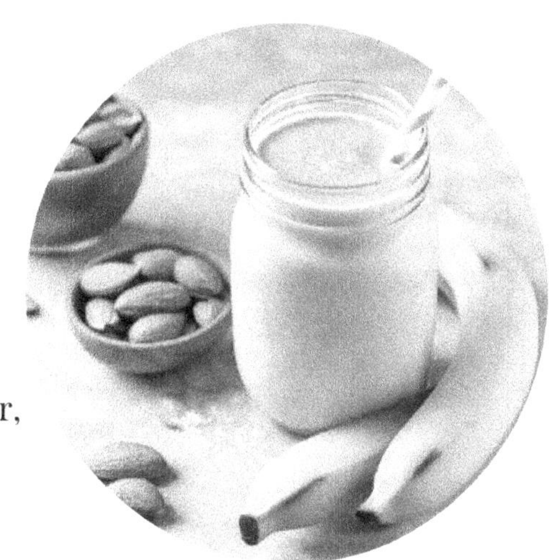

This Almond Butter Banana Smoothie is a satisfying blend of protein-rich almond butter, bananas, and oats, perfect for a quick and nutritious breakfast.

Servings: 1 | Prep Time: 5 minutes | Carbs per Serving: 30g

INGREDIENTS

- 1 banana
- 2 tbsp almond butter (unsweetened)
- 1/4 cup rolled oats
- 1 cup unsweetened almond milk
- 1 tsp cinnamon
- Ice cubes (optional)
- Stevia or honey (optional for added sweetness)

DIRECTIONS

1. In a blender, combine banana, almond butter, rolled oats, almond milk, cinnamon, and ice cubes.
2. Blend until smooth and creamy.
3. Taste and sweeten with stevia or honey if desired.
4. Pour into a glass and enjoy immediately.

NUTRIENT CONTENT (PER SERVING):

- Calories: 300
- Total Fat: 15g
- Protein: 7g
- Carbohydrates: 30g
- Sugars: 10g
- Fiber: 6g
- Sodium: 150mg

HELPFUL INFO:

- Almond Butter: Adds protein and healthy fats, promoting satiety and providing a creamy texture to the smoothie.
- Rolled Oats: High in fiber and complex carbs, oats contribute to stable blood sugar levels and lasting energy.

Family Dinner

Welcome to the heart of the kitchen, where family gatherings and shared meals are transformed into delicious and diabetes-friendly experiences. In the "Pre-Diabetic Diet Cookbook and Meal Plan After 50," this chapter is dedicated to providing you with wholesome and flavorful dinner recipes that cater to managing pre-diabetes and promoting overall well-being for your entire family.

Family dinners hold a special place in our lives, not just for nourishment but also for fostering connections and creating cherished memories. With a focus on balancing glucose levels and preventing prediabetes, these recipes are carefully crafted to be both nutritious and satisfying for everyone at the table.

In this chapter, you'll discover a diverse range of dinner ideas that incorporate lean proteins, fiber-rich vegetables, and complex carbohydrates. From comforting stews and hearty salads to flavorful poultry and fish dishes, each recipe is designed to support stable blood sugar levels while delighting your taste buds.

Whether you're cooking for a small family gathering or hosting a larger dinner party, these family dinner recipes are adaptable, delicious, and suitable for individuals managing pre-diabetes or diabetes. Get ready to create memorable moments around the dinner table with meals that nourish and support your health goals.

Let's embark on a culinary journey that brings joy, connection, and wellness to your family dinners.

COCONUT-CRUSTED BAKED TILAPIA

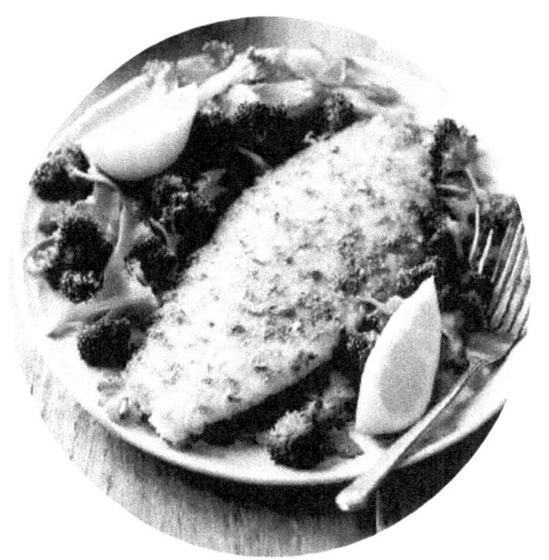

Coconut adds a tropical flavor and healthy fats to the dish while keeping the carb content low.

Servings: 4 | Prep Time: 10 minutes | Cook Time: 15 minutes | Carbs per Serving: 5g

INGREDIENTS

- 4 tilapia fillets
- 1/2 cup shredded unsweetened coconut
- 1/4 cup almond flour
- 1 teaspoon garlic powder
- 1 teaspoon paprika
- Salt and pepper to taste
- 2 eggs, beaten
- Cooking spray or olive oil

DIRECTIONS

1. Preheat the oven to 400°F (200°C). Line a baking sheet with parchment paper and lightly grease with cooking spray or olive oil.
2. In a shallow dish, combine shredded coconut, almond flour, garlic powder, paprika, salt, and pepper.
3. Dip each tilapia fillet into the beaten eggs, ensuring they are evenly coated.
4. Dredge the egg-coated fillets in the coconut mixture, pressing gently to coat both sides.
5. Place the coated tilapia fillets on the prepared baking sheet.
6. Bake in the preheated oven for about 12–15 minutes or until the fish flakes easily with a fork and the coconut coating is golden brown.
7. Remove from the oven and serve the coconut-crusted tilapia hot.

NUTRIENT CONTENT (PER SERVING):	HELPFUL INFO:
<ul><li>Calories: 220</li><li>Total Fat: 11g</li><li>Protein: 26g</li><li>Carbohydrates: 5g</li><li>Sugars: 1g</li><li>Fiber: 2g</li><li>Sodium: 90mg</li></ul>	<ul><li>Tilapia is a lean protein source that's low in saturated fat and high in essential nutrients like omega-3 fatty acids.</li><li>Coconut adds a tropical flavor and healthy fats to the dish while keeping the carb content low.</li><li>Baking instead of frying reduces the overall fat content and makes this dish diabetes-friendly.</li></ul>

QUINOA STUFFED BELL PEPPERS

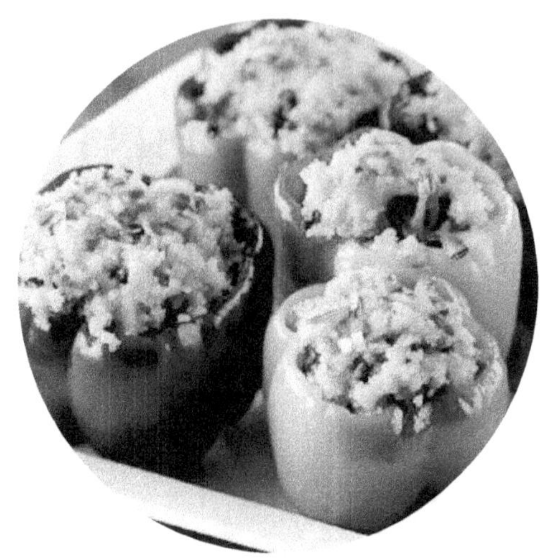

A low-glycemic index grain that provides complex carbohydrates, fiber, and protein, making it a great choice for managing blood sugar

Servings: 4 | Prep Time: 15 minutes | Cook Time: 25 minutes | Carbs per Serving: 35g

INGREDIENTS

- 4 large bell peppers (any color)
- 1 cup cooked quinoa
- 1 cup black beans, drained and rinsed
- 1 cup diced tomatoes
- 1/2 cup corn kernels
- 1/2 cup chopped onion
- 1/2 cup chopped bell peppers (from tops of large bell peppers)
- 1/2 teaspoon cumin
- 1/2 teaspoon chili powder
- Salt and pepper to taste
- 1 cup shredded cheese (optional)
- Fresh cilantro for garnish

DIRECTIONS

1. Preheat the oven to 375°F (190°C). Grease a baking dish with olive oil or cooking spray.
2. Cut the tops off the bell peppers and remove the seeds and membranes. Chop the tops and set aside.
3. In a large mixing bowl, combine cooked quinoa, black beans, diced tomatoes, corn kernels, chopped onion, chopped bell peppers, cumin, chili powder, salt, and pepper. Mix well to combine.
4. Stuff the mixture into the hollowed-out bell peppers and place them in the prepared baking dish.
5. If using cheese, sprinkle shredded cheese on top of each stuffed pepper.
6. Cover the baking dish with aluminum foil and bake in the preheated oven for about 20-25 minutes or until the peppers are tender.
7. Remove the foil and bake for an additional 5 minutes to melt the cheese (if using).
8. Garnish with fresh cilantro before serving.

NUTRIENT CONTENT (PER SERVING):	HELPFUL INFO:
<ul><li>Calories: 300</li><li>Total Fat: 8g</li><li>Protein: 12g</li><li>Carbohydrates: 35g</li><li>Sugars: 5g</li><li>Fiber: 8g</li><li>Sodium: 350mg</li></ul>	<ul><li>Quinoa is a low-glycemic index grain that provides complex carbohydrates, fiber, and protein, making it a great choice for managing blood sugar.</li><li>Black beans are rich in fiber and protein, which helps stabilize blood sugar levels.</li><li>Opt for reduced-fat cheese or omit it entirely</li></ul>

VEGGIE HUMMUS WRAP

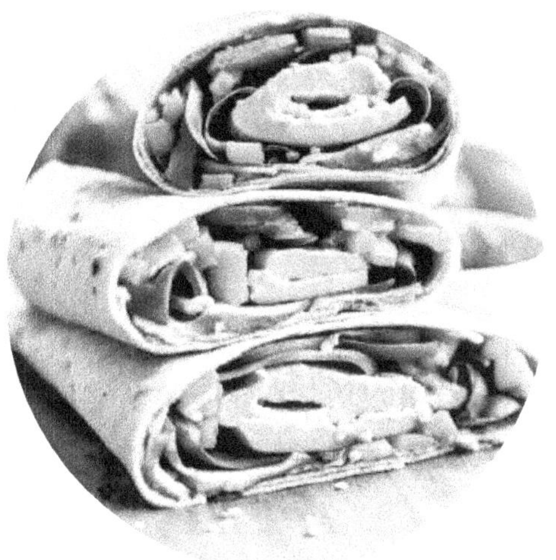

Healthy fats, protein, and fiber, making it a satisfying and blood sugar-friendly spread.

Servings: 4 | Prep Time: 15 minutes | Cook Time: 0 minutes | Carbs per Serving: 30g

INGREDIENTS

- 4 whole-grain wraps or tortillas
- 1 cup hummus
- 1 cup mixed salad greens
- 1/2 cup sliced cucumber
- 1/2 cup shredded carrots
- 1/2 cup sliced bell peppers (any color)
- 1/4 cup sliced red onion
- 1/4 cup crumbled feta cheese (optional)
- 1 tablespoon olive oil
- 1 tablespoon lemon juice
- Salt and pepper to taste

DIRECTIONS

1. In a small bowl, whisk together olive oil, lemon juice, salt, and pepper to make a dressing.
2. Lay out the whole-grain wraps or tortillas on a flat surface.
3. Spread hummus evenly over each wrap, leaving a border around the edges.
4. In the center of each wrap, layer mixed salad greens, sliced cucumber, shredded carrots, sliced bell peppers, and red onion.
5. Drizzle the prepared dressing over the veggies.
6. If using, sprinkle crumbled feta cheese on top of the veggies.
7. Roll up the wraps tightly, folding in the sides as you go, to create a secure wrap.
8. Slice the wraps in half diagonally and serve immediately, or wrap them in foil for later.

NUTRIENT CONTENT (PER SERVING):	HELPFUL INFO:
<ul><li>Calories: 280</li><li>Total Fat: 10g</li><li>Protein: 8g</li><li>Carbohydrates: 30g</li><li>Sugars: 4g</li><li>Fiber: 6g</li><li>Sodium: 450mg</li></ul>	<ul><li>Choose whole-grain wraps or tortillas to increase fiber content and slow down digestion, which can help prevent blood sugar spikes.</li><li>Hummus provides healthy fats, protein, and fiber, making it a satisfying and blood sugar-friendly spread.</li><li>Load up on colorful vegetables for a variety of nutrients and antioxidants without adding excessive carbs.</li></ul>

ASIAN CHICKEN NOODLE SOUP

Healthy fats, protein, and fiber, making it a satisfying and blood sugar-friendly spread.

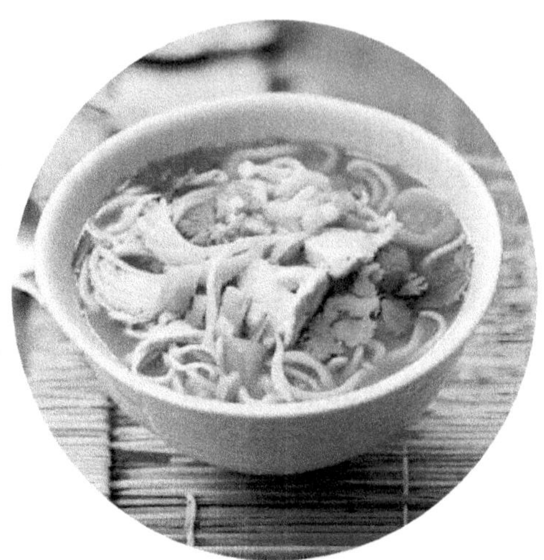

Servings: 6 | Prep Time: 10 minutes | Cook Time: 20 minutes | Carbs per Serving: 30g

INGREDIENTS

- 8 cups low-sodium chicken broth
- 2 boneless, skinless chicken breasts
- 8 oz whole wheat spaghetti or rice noodles
- 1 cup sliced mushrooms
- 1 cup sliced carrots
- 1 cup chopped bok choy or spinach
- 1/4 cup soy sauce (reduced sodium)
- 2 tablespoons fresh ginger, grated
- 2 garlic cloves, minced
- 1 tablespoon sesame oil
- Salt and pepper to taste
- Green onions for garnish

DIRECTIONS

1. In a large pot, bring the chicken broth to a boil.
2. Add chicken breasts to the boiling broth and simmer for about 15-20 minutes until cooked through. Remove chicken and shred with two forks.
3. In the same pot, add noodles, mushrooms, carrots, bok choy/spinach, soy sauce, ginger, garlic, sesame oil, salt, and pepper. Cook according to noodle package instructions until noodles are tender.
4. Return shredded chicken to the pot and simmer for an additional 5 minutes.
5. Adjust seasoning if needed and ladle the soup into bowls.
6. Garnish with sliced green onions before serving.

NUTRIENT CONTENT (PER SERVING):	HELPFUL INFO:
<ul><li>Calories: 280</li><li>Total Fat: 6g</li><li>Protein: 30g</li><li>Carbohydrates: 30g</li><li>Sugars: 3g</li><li>Fiber: 5g</li><li>Sodium: 800mg</li></ul>	<ul><li>Opt for whole wheat or rice noodles to increase fiber content and slow down glucose absorption.</li><li>Use reduced-sodium soy sauce to lower overall sodium content.</li><li>Load the soup with veggies for added fiber, vitamins, and minerals.</li></ul>

GARLIC HERB GRILLED HALIBUT

Lean protein source that is low in saturated fat and carbs, making it a good option for managing blood sugar level

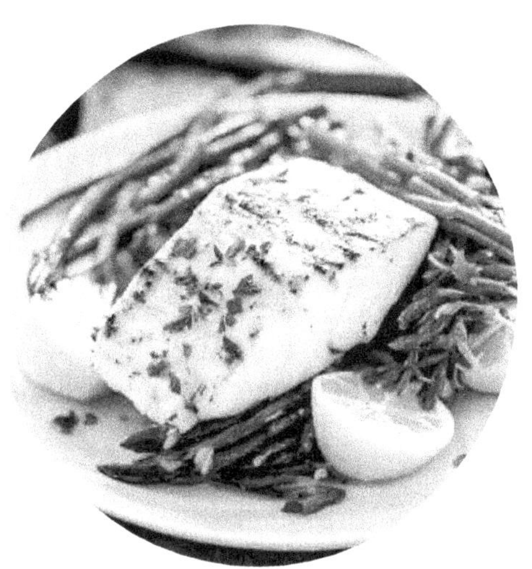

Servings: 4 | Prep Time: 10 minutes | Cook Time: 10 minutes | Carbs per Serving: 1g

INGREDIENTS

- 4 halibut fillets (6 oz each)
- 4 cloves garlic, minced
- 2 tablespoons chopped fresh parsley
- 2 tablespoons chopped fresh dill
- 2 tablespoons olive oil
- 1 lemon, juiced
- Salt and pepper to taste
-

DIRECTIONS

1. In a small bowl, combine minced garlic, chopped parsley, chopped dill, olive oil, lemon juice, salt, and pepper to make the marinade.
2. Place the halibut fillets in a shallow dish and pour the marinade over them, ensuring each fillet is coated evenly. Marinate in the refrigerator for at least 30 minutes.
3. Preheat the grill to medium-high heat and lightly oil the grates to prevent sticking.
4. Remove the halibut fillets from the marinade and place them on the grill. Discard any excess marinade.
5. Grill the halibut for about 4-5 minutes per side, or until the fish is opaque and easily flakes with a fork.
6. Remove the grilled halibut from the heat and let it rest for a few minutes before serving.
7. Serve the garlic herb grilled halibut with your choice of side dishes or a fresh salad.

NUTRIENT CONTENT (PER SERVING):	HELPFUL INFO:
<ul><li>Calories: 240</li><li>Total Fat: 12g</li><li>Protein: 32g</li><li>Carbohydrates: 1g</li><li>Sugars: 0g</li><li>Fiber: 0g</li><li>Sodium: 80mg</li></ul>	<ul><li>Halibut is a lean protein source that is low in saturated fat and carbs, making it a good option for managing blood sugar levels.</li><li>Use fresh herbs and lemon juice to flavor the fish without adding extra sodium or sugar.</li><li>Pair the grilled halibut with non-starchy vegetables or a whole grain side dish for a balanced meal.</li></ul>

SHRIMP AND AVOCADO SALAD

Low-calorie and protein-rich seafood choice that can help manage blood sugar levels.

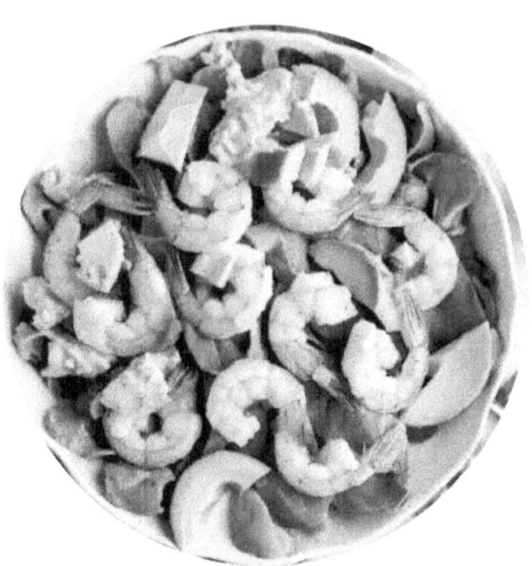

Servings: 4 | Prep Time: 15 minutes | Cook Time: 5 minutes | Carbs per Serving: 8g

INGREDIENTS

- 1 pound shrimp, peeled and deveined
- 2 avocados, diced
- 1 cup cherry tomatoes, halved
- 1/4 cup red onion, finely chopped
- 1/4 cup fresh cilantro, chopped
- 2 tablespoons olive oil
- 2 tablespoons lime juice
- Salt and pepper to taste
- Optional: 1 jalapeño, seeded and diced (for added spice)

DIRECTIONS

1. In a large bowl, combine the diced avocados, cherry tomatoes, red onion, cilantro, and optional jalapeño.
2. In a separate bowl, whisk together olive oil, lime juice, salt, and pepper to make the dressing.
3. Season the shrimp with salt and pepper.
4. Heat a skillet over medium-high heat and add a drizzle of olive oil. Cook the shrimp for about 2-3 minutes per side or until they are pink and opaque.
5. Add the cooked shrimp to the bowl of avocado mixture.
6. Pour the dressing over the salad and gently toss to coat everything evenly.
7. Serve the shrimp and avocado salad immediately as a refreshing and satisfying lunch option.

NUTRIENT CONTENT (PER SERVING):	HELPFUL INFO:
<ul><li>Calories: 320</li><li>Total Fat: 20g</li><li>Protein: 25g</li><li>Carbohydrates: 8g</li><li>Sugars: 2g</li><li>Fiber: 5g</li><li>Sodium: 180mg</li></ul>	<ul><li>Shrimp is a low-calorie and protein-rich seafood choice that can help manage blood sugar levels.</li><li>Avocado adds healthy fats and fiber to the salad, promoting satiety and preventing rapid glucose spikes.</li><li>Use a light dressing with olive oil and lime juice instead of store-bought dressings high in sugar and sodium.</li></ul>

PAN-SEARED TUNA STEAK WITH LEMON HERB BUTTER

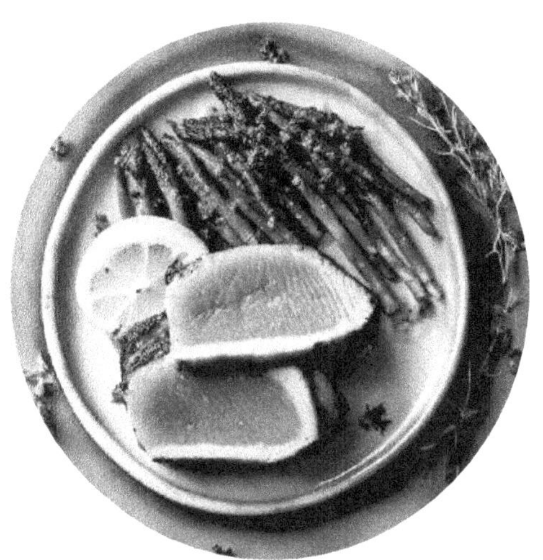

A lean protein source rich in omega-3 fatty acids, which can help improve insulin sensitivity & regulate blood sugar levels.

Servings: 4 | Prep Time: 10 minutes | Cook Time: 8 minutes | Carbs per Serving: 0g

INGREDIENTS

- 4 tuna steaks, about 6 ounces each
- 2 tablespoons olive oil
- Salt and pepper to taste
- 4 tablespoons unsalted butter, softened
- 2 tablespoons fresh parsley, chopped
- 1 tablespoon fresh dill, chopped
- Zest of 1 lemon
- Juice of 1/2 lemon

DIRECTIONS

1. Pat the tuna steaks dry with paper towels and season both sides with salt and pepper.
2. Heat olive oil in a skillet over medium-high heat.
3. Add the tuna steaks to the skillet and sear for about 2-3 minutes per side for medium-rare, or adjust cooking time to your desired doneness.
4. While the tuna is cooking, prepare the lemon herb butter. In a small bowl, combine softened butter, chopped parsley, chopped dill, lemon zest, and lemon juice. Mix until well combined.
5. Once the tuna steaks are cooked to your liking, remove them from the skillet and place them on a serving plate.
6. Top each tuna steak with a generous dollop of lemon herb butter.
7. Allow the butter to melt slightly over the warm tuna steaks before serving.

NUTRIENT CONTENT (PER SERVING):	HELPFUL INFO:
<ul><li>Calories: 300</li><li>Total Fat: 18g</li><li>Protein: 32g</li><li>Carbohydrates: 0g</li><li>Sugars: 0g</li><li>Fiber: 0g</li><li>Sodium: 180mg</li></ul>	<ul><li>Tuna, a lean protein source rich in omega-3 fatty acids, which can help improve insulin sensitivity & regulate blood sugar levels.</li><li>Lemon herb butter adds flavor without adding carbohydrates, making it a diabetic-friendly option.</li><li>Pair this dish with a side of non-starchy vegetables or a small portion of whole grains to create a balanced and nutritious meal.</li></ul>

GRILLED LEMON HERB CHICKEN WITH QUINOA AND STEAMED BROCCOLI

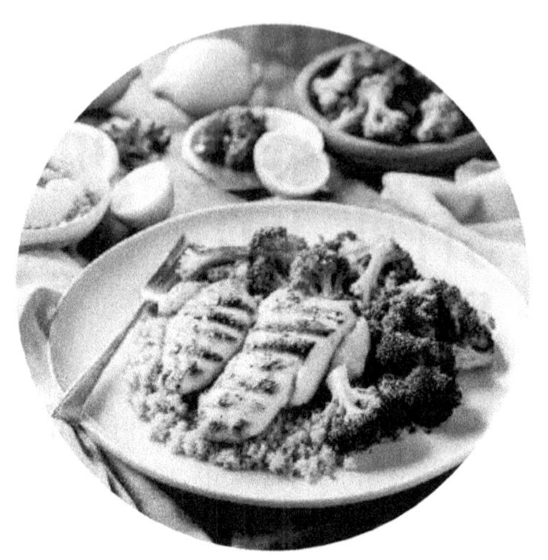

A simple and flavorful dinner that's perfect for any night of the week. The grilled lemon herb chicken pairs wonderfully with nutrient-dense quinoa and steamed broccoli.

Servings: 4 | Prep Time: 30 minutes (plus marinating) | Cook Time: 30 minutes | Carbs per Serving: 25g

INGREDIENTS

- Chicken: 4 boneless, skinless chicken breasts
- Marinade:
  - Juice of 2 lemons
  - 2 tbsp olive oil
  - 3 cloves garlic, minced
  - 1 tsp dried oregano
  - Salt and pepper to taste
- Quinoa: 1 cup quinoa
- Broccoli: 2 cups broccoli florets

DIRECTIONS

1. Marinate Chicken: In a bowl, mix lemon juice, olive oil, garlic, oregano, salt, and pepper. Add chicken breasts and marinate for at least 30 minutes.
2. Cook Quinoa: Rinse quinoa. In a pot, combine quinoa with 2 cups of water. Bring to a boil, then reduce to a simmer and cook for 15 minutes or until water is absorbed.
3. Grill Chicken: Preheat grill to medium-high heat. Grill chicken for 6-7 minutes per side, or until fully cooked.
4. Steam Broccoli: Steam broccoli florets for about 5-7 minutes until tender.
5. Serve: Plate grilled chicken with quinoa and steamed broccoli.

NUTRIENT CONTENT (PER SERVING):	HELPFUL INFO:
<ul><li>Calories: 350</li><li>Total Fat: 12g</li><li>Protein: 30g</li><li>Carbohydrates: 25g</li><li>Sugars: 3g</li><li>Fiber: 5g</li><li>Sodium: 220mg</li></ul>	<ul><li>Chicken: Lean protein that helps maintain muscle mass and keep you full.</li><li>Quinoa: A complex carb with a low glycemic index, high in protein and fiber.</li><li>Broccoli: High in fiber and essential vitamins, helping to manage blood sugar levels.</li></ul>

BAKED SALMON WITH ASPARAGUS AND BROWN RICE

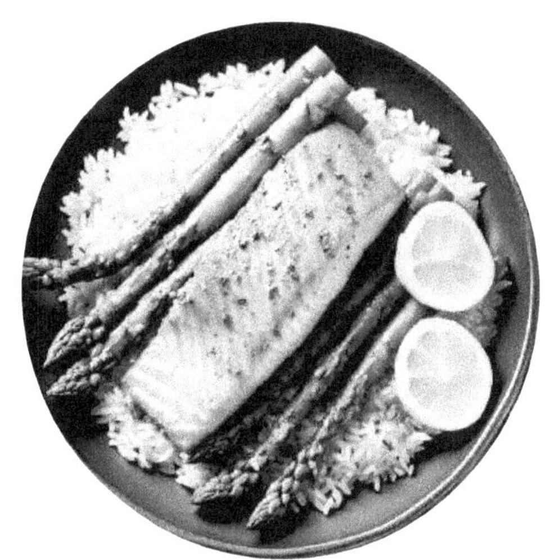

This heart-healthy dinner combines omega-3 rich salmon with fiber-packed brown rice and nutrient-dense asparagus.

Servings: 4 | Prep Time: 10 minutes | Cook Time: 45 minutes | Carbs per Serving: 35g

INGREDIENTS

- Salmon: 4 salmon fillets
- Seasoning:
    - 2 tbsp olive oil
    - 1 tbsp fresh dill, chopped
    - 1 lemon, sliced
    - Salt and pepper to taste
- Asparagus: 1 lb asparagus, trimmed
- Brown Rice: 1 cup brown rice

DIRECTIONS

1. Preheat Oven: Preheat oven to 375°F (190°C).
2. Prepare Salmon: Place salmon fillets on a baking sheet. Drizzle with olive oil, sprinkle with dill, and top with lemon slices. Season with salt and pepper.
3. Bake Salmon: Bake for 20-25 minutes until salmon is cooked through.
4. Cook Brown Rice: In a pot, combine brown rice with 2 cups of water. Bring to a boil, then reduce to a simmer and cook for 45 minutes or until water is absorbed.
5. Steam Asparagus: Steam asparagus for 5-7 minutes until tender.
6. Serve: Plate salmon with brown rice and asparagus.

NUTRIENT CONTENT (PER SERVING):	HELPFUL INFO:
<ul><li>Calories: 400</li><li>Total Fat: 18g</li><li>Protein: 30g</li><li>Carbohydrates: 35g</li><li>Sugars: 2g</li><li>Fiber: 6g</li><li>Sodium: 200mg</li></ul>	<ul><li>Salmon: Rich in omega-3 fatty acids, which support heart health.</li><li>Brown Rice: A whole grain with a low glycemic index, providing sustained energy.</li><li>Asparagus: Contains fiber and antioxidants, helping to regulate blood sugar levels.</li></ul>

SPAGHETTI SQUASH WITH TOMATO BASIL SAUCE

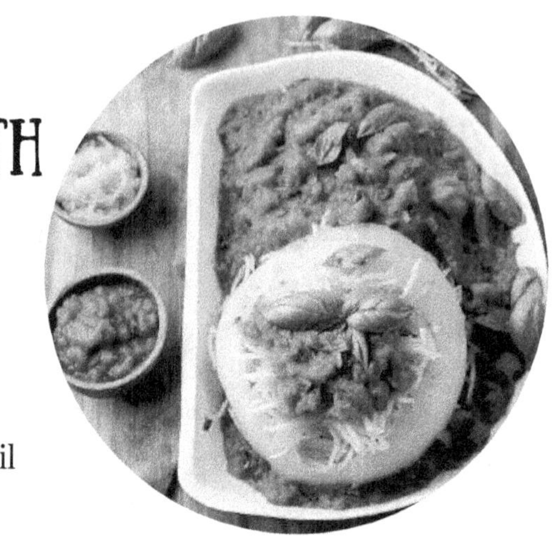

A low-carb alternative to pasta, spaghetti squash paired with a homemade tomato basil sauce offers a satisfying and healthy dinner option.

Servings: 4 | Prep Time: 10 minutes | Cook Time: 40 minutes | Carbs per Serving: 20g

INGREDIENTS

- Spaghetti Squash: 1 large spaghetti squash
- Sauce:
  - 2 tbsp olive oil
  - 1 onion, chopped
  - 2 cloves garlic, minced
  - 4 tomatoes, chopped
  - 1 tsp dried basil
  - Salt and pepper to taste

DIRECTIONS

1. Preheat Oven: Preheat oven to 400°F (200°C).
2. Cook Squash: Cut spaghetti squash in half lengthwise and remove seeds. Drizzle with olive oil, season with salt and pepper, and place cut side down on a baking sheet. Roast for 40 minutes.
3. Make Sauce: In a skillet, heat olive oil over medium heat. Add onion and garlic, cooking until softened. Add tomatoes and basil, simmering for 15 minutes.
4. Prepare Squash: Remove squash from the oven and use a fork to scrape out the flesh into spaghetti-like strands.
5. Serve: Plate spaghetti squash and top with tomato basil sauce.

NUTRIENT CONTENT (PER SERVING):	HELPFUL INFO:
• Calories: 200 • Total Fat: 10g • Protein: 3g • Carbohydrates: 20g • Sugars: 10g • Fiber: 5g • Sodium: 150mg	• Spaghetti Squash: Low in carbohydrates and high in fiber, making it a great pasta substitute. • Tomatoes: Rich in antioxidants and vitamins. • Basil: Adds flavor and nutrients without adding extra calories.

Prediabetes Meal Plan and Grocery List

Embarking on a journey to manage prediabetes through diet can feel overwhelming, but it doesn't have to be. The "Prediabetes Meal Plan and Grocery List" chapter is designed to simplify the process and guide you step-by-step towards a healthier lifestyle. This chapter provides a comprehensive 21-day meal plan tailored specifically for women over 50, focusing on balanced meals that stabilize blood sugar levels, promote weight management, and support overall well-being.

When it comes to managing prediabetes, what you eat plays a pivotal role. The meal plan in this chapter emphasizes nutrient-dense foods, rich in fiber, lean protein, healthy fats, and complex carbohydrates. You'll find a variety of delicious recipes that incorporate green vegetables, which are known for their blood sugar-regulating properties. These recipes are not only nutritious but also flavorful, ensuring that you enjoy every meal while keeping your health in check.

In addition to the meal plan, this chapter includes a detailed grocery list. This list is your roadmap to efficient and effective shopping, ensuring you have all the ingredients needed for your prediabetes-friendly meals. From fresh produce to pantry staples, the list covers everything required to prepare breakfasts, lunches, dinners, and snacks for the entire three weeks.

To maximize the benefits of your diet, it's important to understand the role of different types of carbohydrates. Opting for complex carbs and pairing them with other nutrients can significantly impact how your body processes sugar. Think of it as dressing up your carbs to keep your glucose levels steady and happy.

Whether you are looking to prevent the onset of type 2 diabetes or manage your current prediabetes condition, this meal plan and grocery list are invaluable tools. They provide structure, variety, and practicality, making it easier to adopt and maintain a healthy eating pattern. Dive into this chapter, and take the first steps towards a healthier, more balanced life.

WEEK 1: PREDIABETES MEAL PLAN

	BREAKFAST	LUNCH	DINNER	SNACKS
MON	Spinach and Mushroom Frittata	Chicken and Quinoa Salad with Lemon Vinaigrette	Almond Butter Banana Smoothie	Grilled Lemon Herb Chicken with Quinoa and Steamed Broccoli
TUES	Chia Seed Pudding with Berries	Quinoa and Black Bean Stuffed Peppers	Avocado Yogurt Dip with Veggie Sticks	Baked Salmon with Asparagus and Brown Rice
WED	Avocado Toast with Poached Egg	Mediterranean Chickpea Salad	Berry Bliss Delight Smoothie	Lentil and Mushroom Shepherd's Pie
THURS	Greek Yogurt Parfait with Nuts and Seeds	Shrimp and Avocado Salad	Spicy Sriracha Mayo with Veggie Sticks	Lemon Garlic Roast Chicken Thighs with Steamed Veggies
FRI	Quinoa Breakfast Bowl	Chicken and Vegetable Soup	Berry Avocado Powerhouse Smoothie	Coconut-Crusted Baked Tilapia
SAT	Sweet Potato Hash	Lentil Vegetable Soup	Roasted Red Pepper Hummus with Veggie Sticks	Baked Cod with Roasted Vegetables
SUN	Berry Almond Smoothie	Eggplant and Tomato Stew	Creamy Garlic Parmesan Dip with Veggie Sticks	Beef and Vegetable Stir-Fry with Quinoa

WEEK 2:PREDIABETES MEAL PLAN

	BREAKFAST	LUNCH	DINNER	SNACKS
MON	Greek Yogurt and Berry Parfait	Turkey and Vegetable Stir-Fry	Spinach Berry Blast Smoothie	Mediterranean Grilled Swordfish with Steamed Veggies
TUES	Oatmeal with Walnuts and Pear	Stuffed Acorn Squash with Quinoa and Cranberries	Tropical Mango Tango Smoothie	Spaghetti Squash with Tomato Basil Sauce
WED	Veggie Scramble with Avocado	Roasted Cauliflower and Chickpea Curry	Tangy Honey Mustard Dip with Veggie Sticks	Grilled Salmon with Lemon Herb Butter and Steamed Veggies
THURS	Almond Flour Pancakes with Blueberry Sauce	Chicken and Spinach Alfredo Pasta	Tropical Turmeric Delight Smoothie	Shrimp and Avocado Salad
FRI	Tomato and Zucchini Omelette	Barley and Roasted Vegetable Pilaf	Tangy Balsamic Vinaigrette with Veggie Sticks	Beef Stir-Fry with Broccoli and Brown Rice
SAT	Cottage Cheese and Peach Bowl	Eggplant Parmesan	Chocolate Peanut Butter Bliss Smoothie	Lemon Herb Roasted Chicken Breast with Steamed Veggies
SUN	Kale and White Bean Breakfast Sauté	Zucchini Noodles with Pesto and Cherry Tomatoes	Cinnamon Apple Pie Delight Smoothie	Lamb Curry with Cauliflower Rice

WEEK 3:PREDIABETES MEAL PLAN

	BREAKFAST	LUNCH	DINNER	SNACKS
MON	Broccoli and Cheese Egg Muffins	Mediterranean Veggie Omelette	Green Power Smoothie	Pan-Seared Tuna Steak with Lemon Herb Butter
TUES	Cinnamon Almond Porridge	Chickpea and Spinach Curry	Lemon Herb Yogurt Sauce with Veggie Sticks	Turkey and Lentil Stuffed Bell Peppers
WED	Smoked Salmon and Avocado Wrap	Vegetable Paella	Berry Blast Smoothie	Coconut Lime Shrimp Curry
THURS	Mediterranean Veggie Omelette	Caprese Stuffed Portobello Mushrooms	Avocado Lime Dressing with Veggie Sticks	Turkey and Vegetable Skewers with Steamed Veggies
FRI	Pumpkin Seed and Almond Yogurt	Autumn Bisque	Tropical Paradise Smoothie	Garlic Herb Grilled Halibut with Steamed Veggies
SAT	Avocado and Egg Breakfast Salad	Tomato and White Bean Stew	Creamy Cilantro Lime Dressing with Veggie Sticks	Baked Lemon Herb Tilapia with Steamed Veggies
SUN	Greek Yogurt Parfait with Nuts and Seeds	Chickpea and Vegetable Stir-Fry	Roasted Red Pepper Hummus with Veggie Sticks	Grilled Lemon Herb Turkey Cutlets with Steamed Veggies

GROCERY SHOPPING LIST FOR PREDIABETES MEAL PLAN

MEAT & SEAFOOD

Chicken breasts: 6 lbs
Chicken thighs: 4 lbs
Turkey breast cutlets: 3 lbs
Ground turkey: 3 lbs
Shrimp: 3 lbs

Lamb chops: 2 lbs
Pork tenderloin: 2 lbs
Pork chops: 4
Cod fillets: 3 lbs
Salmon fillets: 4 lbs

Tuna steaks: 2 lbs
Swordfish: 2 lbs
Tilapia fillets: 2 lbs
Ground beef: 2 lbs
Beef stir-fry strips: 2 lbs

GRAINS & LEGUMES

Quinoa: 5 cups
Barley: 2 cups
Brown rice: 4 cups
Whole wheat bread: 2 loaves
Whole wheat tortillas: 1 pack

Steel-cut oats: 4 cups
Chia seeds: 2 cups
Almond flour: 2 lbs
Walnuts: 2 cups
Almonds: 3 cups

Lentils: 4 cups
Black beans: 3 cups
Chickpeas: 5 cups
White beans: 3 cups
Pumpkin seeds: 1 cup

DAIRY AND EGGS

Eggs: 4 dozen
Greek yogurt (plain, unsweetened): 14 cups

Cottage cheese: 2 cups
Almond milk (unsweetened): 4 quarts
Parmesan cheese: 1 cup

Cheddar cheese: 4 cups
Feta cheese: 2 cups
Mozzarella cheese: 2 cups

CANNED & JARRED GOODS

Balsamic vinegar: 1 bottle
Olive oil: 1 bottle
Maple syrup: 1 bottle
Sriracha: 1 bottle

Diced tomatoes: 10 cans (15 oz each)
Tomato sauce: 4 cans (15 oz each)
Tomato paste: 2 cans (6 oz each)
Coconut milk: 6 cans (15 oz each)

Soy sauce (low sodium): 1 bottle
Honey: 1 bottle
Peanut butter: 1 jar (16 oz)
Hummus: 2 containers (16 oz each)

Avocados: 12
Bananas: 8
Apples: 6
Pears: 3
Peaches: 2
Lemons: 8
Limes: 6
Zucchini: 15
Cucumbers: 6
Sweet potatoes: 6
Spaghetti squash: 3
Acorn squash: 2
Carrots: 4 lbs

Mushrooms: 4 lbs
Blueberries: 4 cups
Raspberries: 4 cups
Strawberries: 4 cups
Ginger: 1 large piece
Tomatoes: 12
Cherry tomatoes: 6 cups
Bell peppers (various colors): 24
Spinach: 5 bags (10 oz each)
Mixed greens: 4 bags (10 oz each)

Fresh herbs (basil, cilantro, parsley, mint, rosemary, thyme): 1 bunch each

Celery: 3 bunches
Kale: 3 bunches
Broccoli: 4 heads
Cauliflower: 4 heads
Brussels sprouts: 2 lbs
Garlic: 3 bulbs
Red onions: 6
Yellow onions: 12
Eggplant: 5
Butternut squash: 2
Green onions: 3 bunches
Asparagus: 4 bunches

SPICES AND SEASONINGS

Salt
Black pepper
Cumin
Paprika

Turmeric
Chili powder
Cinnamon
Nutmeg

Italian seasoning
Curry powder
Garlic powder
Onion powder
Red pepper flakes

MISCELLANEOUS

Baking powder: 1 small container

Baking soda: 1 small container

Vanilla extract: 1 small bottle

Appendix 1: Measurement Conversions

Volume Equivalents (Liquid)

US STANDARD	US STANDARD (OUNCES)	METRIC (APPROXIMATE)
2 tablespoons	1 fl. oz.	30 mL
¼ cup	2 fl. oz.	60 mL
½ cup	4 fl. oz.	120 mL
1 cup	8 fl. oz.	240 mL
1½ cups	12 fl. oz.	355 mL
2 cups or 1 pint	16 fl. oz.	475 mL
4 cups or 1 quart	32 fl. oz.	1 L
1 gallon	128 fl. oz.	4 L

Volume Equivalents (Dry)

US STANDARD	METRIC (APPROXIMATE)
⅛ teaspoon	0.5 mL
¼ teaspoon	1 mL
½ teaspoon	2 mL
¾ teaspoon	4 mL
1 teaspoon	5 mL
1 tablespoon	15 mL
¼ cup	59 mL
⅓ cup	79 mL
½ cup	118 mL
⅔ cup	156 mL
¾ cup	177 mL
1 cup	235 mL
2 cups or 1 pint	475 mL
3 cups	700 mL
4 cups or 1 quart	1 L

Oven Temperatures

FAHRENHEIT	CELSIUS (APPROXIMATE)
250°F	120°C
300°F	150°C
325°F	165°C
350°F	180°C
375°F	190°C
400°F	200°C
425°F	220°C
450°F	230°C

Weight Equivalents

FAHRENHEIT	CELSIUS (APPROXIMATE)
½ ounce	15g
1 ounce	30g
2 ounces	60g
4 ounces	115g
8 ounces	225g
12 ounces	340g
16 ounces or 1 pound	455g

Appendix 2: The 2024 Dirty Dozen™ and Clean Fifteen™

The Dirty Dozen and the Clean Fifteen™ refer to lists compiled by the Environmental Working Group (EWG), an organization dedicated to environmental health. They analyze data from the USDA and FDA regarding pesticide residues in commercial crops. These lists help consumers make informed choices about buying organic versus conventional produce based on pesticide levels.

The Dirty Dozen includes fruits and vegetables with the highest pesticide loads, while the Clean Fifteen™ comprises produce with lower pesticide residues. It's essential to note that even items on the Clean Fifteen™ may still have pesticide residues, so thorough washing is advised.

Since these lists are updated annually, it's crucial to check the latest version before grocery shopping.
Visit www.ewg.org/FoodNews for the most recent lists and a comprehensive guide to pesticides in produce.

DIRTY DOZEN™	CLEAN FIFTEEN™
◯ Strawberries	◯ Carrots
◯ Spinach	◯ Sweet Potatoes
◯ Kale, collard & mustard greens	◯ Mangoes
◯ Grapes	◯ Mushrooms
◯ Peaches	◯ Watermelon
◯ Pears	◯ Cabbage
◯ Nectarines	◯ Kiwi
◯ Apples	◯ Honeydew melon
◯ Bell & hot Peppers	◯ Asparagus
◯ Cherries	◯ Sweet peas (frozen)
◯ Blueberries	◯ Papaya*
◯ Green Beans	◯ Onions
	◯ Pineapple
	◯ Sweet corn*
	◯ Avocados

Appendix 3: Recipe Index

A

- Almond Butter Banana Smoothie, 131
- Almond Flour Pancakes with Blueberry Sauce, 31
- Asian Chicken Noodle Soup, 136
- Autumn Bisque, 57
- Avocado and Egg Breakfast Salad, 40
- Avocado and Turkey Wrap, 75
- Avocado Lime Dressing, 113
- Avocado Toast with Poached Egg, 23
- Avocado Yogurt Dip, 117

B

- Baked Cod with Roasted Vegetables, 107
- Baked Lemon Herb Tilapia, 109
- Baked Salmon with Asparagus and Brown Rice, 141
- Balsamic Roasted Brussels Sprouts, 47
- Barley and Roasted Vegetable Pilaf, 50
- Beef and Vegetable Skewers with Quinoa, 97
- Beef and Vegetable Stir-Fry with Quinoa, 90
- Beef Stir-Fry with Broccoli and Brown Rice, 94
- BEEF, PORK, AND LAMB, 88
- Berry Almond Smoothie, 27
- Berry Avocado Powerhouse, 125
- Berry Blast Smoothie, 129
- Berry Bliss Delight, 121
- Breakfast and Brunch, 20
- Broccoli and Cheese Egg Muffins, 35
- Butternut Squash and Apple Soup, 59

C

- Caprese Salad, 71
- Caprese Stuffed Portobello Mushrooms, 72
- Cauliflower and Chickpea Tacos, 67
- Chia Seed Pudding with Berries, 22
- Chicken and Barley Soup, 56
- Chicken and Quinoa Salad with Lemon Vinaigrette, 84
- Chicken and Spinach Alfredo Pasta, 79
- Chicken and Spinach Stuffed Portobello Mushrooms, 76
- Chicken and Turkey, 74
- Chicken and Vegetable Soup, 60
- Chickpea and Spinach Curry, 52
- Chickpea and Spinach Curry, 65
- Chocolate Peanut Butter Bliss, 127
- Cinnamon Almond Porridge, 36
- Cinnamon Apple Pie Delight, 124
- Coconut Lime Shrimp Curry, 103
- Coconut-Crusted Baked Tilapia, 133
- Cottage Cheese and Peach Bowl, 33
- Creamy Cilantro Lime Dressing, 116
- Creamy Garlic Parmesan Dip, 112
- Creamy Garlic Shrimp Pasta, 100

E

- Eggplant and Tofu Stir-Fry, 46
- Eggplant and Tomato Stew, 66
- Eggplant Parmesan, 70

F

- Family Dinner, 132
- FISH AND SEAFOOD, 99

G

- Garlic Herb Grilled Halibut, 137
- Greek Yogurt and Berry Parfait, 28
- Greek Yogurt Parfait with Nuts and Seeds, 24
- Green Power Smoothie, 128
- Greens and Beans Turkey Soup, 58
- Grilled Lamb Chops with Mint Chimichurri, 92
- Grilled Lemon Herb Chicken with Quinoa and Steamed Broccoli, 140
- Grilled Lemon Herb Turkey Cutlets, 83
- Grilled Salmon with Lemon Herb Butter, 105

K

- Kale and White Bean Breakfast Sauté, 34

L

- Lamb and Chickpea Curry, 96
- Lamb Curry with Cauliflower Rice, 89
- Lemon Garlic Chicken and Broccoli Stir-Fry, 86
- Lemon Garlic Herb Grilled Shrimp, 108
- Lemon Garlic Roast Chicken Thighs, 78
- Lemon Garlic Roasted Asparagus, 49
- Lemon Herb Baked Cod, 101
- Lemon Herb Roasted Chicken Breast, 81
- Lemon Herb Yogurt Sauce, 115
- Lentil and Mushroom Shepherd's Pie, 43
- Lentil and Vegetable Stir-Fry, 64
- Lentil Vegetable Soup, 54

M

- Meatless Main Dishes, 62
- Mediterranean Chickpea Salad, 69
- Mediterranean Grilled Swordfish, 104
- Mediterranean Turkey Meatballs with Zucchini Noodles, 87
- Mediterranean Veggie Omelette, 38

O

- Oatmeal with Walnuts and Pear, 29

P

- Pan-Seared Tuna Steak with Lemon Herb Butter, 139
- Pork and Bean Chili, 98
- Pork Chops with Balsamic Glaze, 91
- Pork Tenderloin with Maple Glaze, 93
- Pork Tenderloin with Roasted Vegetables, 95
- Pumpkin Seed and Almond Yogurt, 39

Q

- Quinoa and Black Bean Stuffed Peppers, 42
- Quinoa Breakfast Bowl, 25
- Quinoa Stuffed Bell Peppers, 134

R

- Roasted Cauliflower and Chickpea Curry, 44
- Roasted Red Pepper Hummus, 119

S

- SAUCE, DIPS, & DRESSINGS, 110
- Shrimp and Avocado Salad, 106
- Shrimp and Avocado Salad, 138
- Smoked Salmon and Avocado Wrap, 37
- SMOOTHIES, 120
- Soup and Stew, 53
- Spaghetti Squash Pad Thai, 68
- Spaghetti Squash Primavera, 51
- Spaghetti Squash with Tomato Basil Sauce, 142
- Spicy Grilled Shrimp Tacos, 102
- Spicy Sriracha Mayo, 111
- Spinach and Mushroom Frittata, 21
- Spinach and White Bean Soup, 61
- Spinach Berry Blast, 123
- Stuffed Acorn Squash with Quinoa and Cranberries, 48
- Sweet Potato Hash, 26

T

- Tangy Balsamic Vinaigrette, 118
- Tangy Honey Mustard Dip 114,
- Tomato and White Bean Stew, 55
- Tomato and Zucchini Omelette, 32
- Tropical Mango Tango, 126
- Tropical Paradise Smoothie, 130
- Tropical Turmeric Delight, 122
- Turkey and Lentil Stuffed Bell Peppers, 77
- Turkey and Quinoa Stuffed Bell Peppers, 80
- Turkey and Vegetable Skewers, 85
- Turkey and Vegetable Stir-Fry, 82

V

- Vegetable Paella, 73
- Vegetarian Mains and Sides, 41
- Veggie Hummus Wrap, 135
- Veggie Scramble with Avocado, 30

Z

- Zucchini Noodles with Pesto, 63
- Zucchini Noodles with Pesto and Cherry Tomatoes, 45